A Woman's Skin

A **W**_oman's_ **S**_kin_

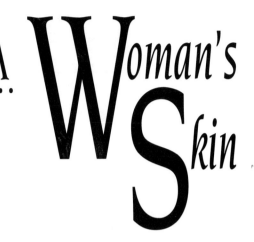

David M. Stoll, M.D.

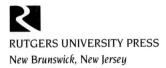

RUTGERS UNIVERSITY PRESS

New Brunswick, New Jersey

Library of Congress Cataloguing-in-Publication Data

    Stoll, David, M.D.
    A woman's skin / David Stoll.
       p.   cm.
    Includes index.
    ISBN 0-8135-2028-2 (cloth)—ISBN 0-8135-2029-0 (pbk.)
    1. Women—Health and hygiene. 2. Women—Diseases. 3. Skin—Care and
hygiene. 4. Skin—Diseases. I. Title.
RL73.W65S76 1994
616.5'0082—dc20
           93-6372
             CIP

British Cataloguing in Publication information available

With Gratitude to Hashem
Dedicated to Dorothy and the Kids

Contents ◀

portwine stains / torn earlobes / excess fat / sagging eyelids / Retin-A / the AHAs / wonder creams that never made it / chemical face peels / dermabrasion / laser treatment / face lifts / liposuction / questions and answers about cosmetic surgery and treatments

A Note of Advice ◄

The material presented in this book is designed to inform you about your skin: how it works, how to take care of it, how it differs from a man's, how to be an educated consumer of skin care and beauty products and of medical treatments, how to recognize signs of skin disease and systemic illnesses that affect the skin, hair, and nails, and how medical treatment can help with allergies, diseases, and cosmetic problems.

However, while I have tried hard to make the information contained in these pages accurate, comprehensive, and up-to-date, this book is not a substitute for a visit to your doctor! The ultimate and best-informed decisions about skin problems must be made in conjunction with a qualified doctor whom you trust.

As a dermatologist, I came to realize the need for medically reliable and balanced information about women and their skin from talking with patients and many other women from all different backgrounds and walks of life. Women's skin *is*, in many important and interesting ways, different from men's skin. But while the medical differences between the sexes has been the subject of countless books, none have been devoted to women's skin. Until now.

It's not that the information isn't out there. In my quest to put this book together, I would find an article here, a news item there, and a section of a book somewhere else. Initially I relied on the dermatology literature and my own clinical experience. But soon I found myself delving into other fields—like obstetrics and gynecology, internal medicine, and nutrition—in order to get the information I increasingly felt to be relevant. My studies even beckoned me into areas physicians do not often consider, like traditional folk treatments and New Age approaches to health and beauty.

At journey's end, the material I had collected represented the basic and the marginal, the popular and the forgotten, the mainstream and the esoteric. I then had to figure out how to pull it together "under one roof," in a book that would be medically sound, comprehensive, and as unbiased as possible. I wanted it to be clear and readable for any woman who wants to know more about her skin. I even hoped I could sometimes make it fun!

I have tried to make this book useful to all women, whatever their age, lifestyle, skin type, race and ethnic background. I've made every attempt to evaluate, from a scientific and clinical point of view, your routine skin care needs and the special skin problems that you, as a woman, may have. Because hair and nails grow out of the skin and share some of its structure, I cover the normal care and the treatment of problems for both.

You need to be able to make sound decisions about which skin care products, cosmetics, and procedures are appropriate for you personally. Every day you are faced with choices: Should you use this cream or that ointment? For this skin problem, should you turn to surgical or to chemical treatments? Solid information about all this is simply hard to find. Much of it comes from manufacturers, the popular media, or word of mouth. Although sometimes it's correct, it isn't always. And it's rarely comprehensive. This can be costly in more ways than one—for skin care and cosmetic practices and products, both the ordinary and the high-tech, have limitations for safety and effectiveness. A good bit of what I cover is meant to help you sift through these issues.

A large part of the book is devoted to the skin care and health issues that come up at different points during your life. The problems you worry about as a teenager are not the same as the ones that you face after menopause—although you can, as a young woman, take simple steps to prevent serious skin problems later in life. I give special attention to skin problems that can occur during pregnancy.

Last but not least, there is the subject of skin reactions (including work-related ones) to allergies and irritants, diseases of the skin, and diseases of the body that affect women's skin. I touch on these throughout the book—check the index—and give a more detailed discussion of many of them in the final chapter. You'll notice, by the way, that the book has no pictures of rashes, bumps, moles, and other signs of skin diseases. That's because a single picture just cannot convey accurately the variety of ways a given skin condition will show up; it might even give you a false sense of reassurance if your problem does not match the picture. If you have a skin condition that concerns you, please check it out with your doctor.

As you read through the book, you will note that not every topic I discuss is unique to women. As a physician, I felt that I would not be giving you good medical information if I failed to cover the whole range of skin health questions that you might encounter. If you learn something here that can help the men in your life as well as yourself, so much the better for everyone.

My ultimate hope is that the information I have supplied will help you understand your skin at various ages of your life, get your skin to look the way you want it to, prevent skin problems and diseases whenever that's possible, and receive the best medical care when you do have difficulties.

Acknowledgments ◀

This book would not have been possible without the knowledge, perspectives, inspiration, and support I received from a wide range of people.

I would like to express my gratitude to Lloyd E. King, Jr., M.D., Ph.D., who guided me through my dermatology residency at Vanderbilt University Medical Center and who encouraged my contribution to the research team that won the Nobel Prize for its work on epidermal growth factor; to James Fields, M.D., Dana Latour, M.D., Lyon Rowe, M.D., Marvin Klapman, M.D., Vince Fowler, M.D., David Goldstein, M.D., and Lamar Nelson, M.D., from whom I always learn so much when we consult with each other on difficult cases in dermatology; and to Faye Kellerman and John Kellerman, who offered me invaluable support and encouragement while I wrote this book.

I also wish to thank the following: Karen Reeds, Science Editor at Rutgers University Press, who went through my manuscript with enormous care and patience, raising important questions and making excellent recommendations; Judith Wisdom, whose editing skills went far beyond issues of language and organization, and included many valuable contributions in matters both scientific and sociological; Robyn Levy, M.D., who did a super job reviewing the manuscript; and Ms. Maryann McCarthy, who put in endless time and effort typing the manuscript and fine-tuning the wording with great sensitivity to the nuances of language.

Special thanks go to innumerable other people, most of them women, from the fields of women's studies, medical history, dermatology, internal medicine, and obstetrics and gynecology, and to women from many other backgrounds and occupations who were kind enough to read the manuscript. They all felt strongly that a medically informed book, written in nonmedical language, about women's skin and the methods available to improve its health and appearance was very much needed. Though we didn't always agree, their comments were extremely helpful to me in my effort to make this book comprehensive and responsive to the needs and problems of the diverse population of women I hope to reach.

I would also like to thank my parents, Dr. and Mrs. Leonard Stoll, and my mother-in-law, Mrs. Zlata Tewel, for their constant support and guidance.

Finally, I want to express my love and appreciation to my wife, Dorothy, and my children, Yaakov, Srully, Goldie, Miriam Baila, Reena, and Yossi, for having put up with a husband and father who spent far too many hours at the typewriter.

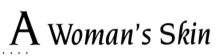

A Woman's Skin

Chapter 1

Women's Skin, Men's Skin— What's the Difference?

A woman's skin is different from a man's. Intuitively, that's what you'd expect, given the number of biological differences between the sexes.

Yet, if you were to look at samples of women's skin and men's skin through a microscope, you would find it hard to tell which was which. The layers are made out of the same kinds of skin cells, the way the hairs grow out of the skin is the same, the sweat and oil glands look the same. You might well see bigger differences in skin samples taken from various parts of one woman's body. Or taken at various ages. Or from one individual to the next. So, what's the difference?

Throughout this book, I will be noting specific differences between women's skin and men's, and what the consequences are for your health and skin care. But I want to start by pointing out the general differences and when and how those differences arise. I find it useful to classify them under three broad categories: structural, sexual, and social. It's in the social and sexual categories where most of the significant practical and functional differences show up.

Structural Differences

When it comes to structure, human skin is much the same, no matter what sex (or race, for that matter) you are. We are, after all, all members of one species, and dermatology textbooks can use one set of diagrams of skin structure for everyone.

Most of us assume that a woman's skin is "delicate" and a man's is "tough." But this depends on how these terms are defined and measured. Studies using ultrasound waves have shown that, at all ages of life, men's skin is thicker than women's.

But when "tougher" is taken to mean how easily skin gets irritated, the results are a bit murkier. Scientific studies have come up with conflicting answers. That's not an uncommon situation in science and medicine, especially at early stages of research, and it's a good reason to be cautious about generalizing from a single study. In this case, one study that looked at skin irritation from certain common chemicals—including soaps and detergents—found no gender-related differences in skin sensitivity to these chemicals. Men and women were equally susceptible. However, another study showed that women *were* more easily irritated by certain chemicals than men were!

Did the researchers in the different studies define or measure susceptibility to irritation differently? Did they use the same chemicals? Were there differences in the skin or lifestyles of the women and men studied that could have accounted for the contradictory results? These are the kinds of questions that science always has to grapple with when devising studies and interpreting results. So, until more studies are reported on this particular issue, the debate will rage on.

Besides thickness and toughness, it is also possible to make comparisons between the sexes with respect to skin extensibility— the ability of the skin to stretch. Both men and women have the same patterns over their lifetime with respect to the skin's ability to stretch—holding steady until the seventh decade, and then becoming less stretchy. Women's skin can show a temporary, but noticeable decrease in extensibility just before a menstrual period.

A very revealing study was conducted in France in 1986 to see if age, sex, or social conditions affected the elasticity of skin— the ability of skin to return to its original size after being stretched. The researchers compared cloistered nuns, white-collar workers, and blue-collar workers. In all three groups, elasticity decreased with age, but in women it had a more rapid rate of decline than it did in men.

Looking just at the two groups of women—the cloistered nuns and the working women—the study found that the group of women who worked outside the home experienced a more rapid decline in skin elasticity than the nuns. Unfortunately, the study could not give a reason for this intriguing result. Was it a difference in work habits, sun exposure, or stress, or what? Until another research project deals specifically with those issues, we simply won't know. (Again, this is very typical of how science moves ahead. Research projects answer certain questions but raise new and interesting ones, which then form the basis for new research projects and new answers.)

Definite differences exist between the sexes with respect to skin temperature. A woman's skin reacts more strongly than a man's to changes in the temperature in the *external* environment. For example, when immersed in cold water, women's skin cools more rapidly than men's. Also, upon exposure to cold air, the average skin temperature of women will be lower than that of men.

What causes a woman's skin to cool more rapidly and to become colder? The current thinking on this is that, since women have a higher percentage of body fat than men do, their skin doesn't have to play as large a role as men's skin does in keeping *their* insides warm.

Another way to put this is that a drop in *skin* temperature alone will have less of an effect on the *internal* temperature of women than it will in men. Women do not need their skin to bear the full brunt of keeping their insides warm. They get help in this "task" from their body fat. Men's skin, by contrast, bears a greater percentage of the burden of keeping their bodies warm, because men have a smaller percentage of body fat.

What about the differences between the sexes in response to heat? Generally, women tolerate heat less well than men do. This means that they are more susceptible to heat stress and to heat stroke. The reason is that women tend to sweat less than men do. As a result, in response to excessive heat, they cannot cool their bodies as rapidly as men can. Therefore, external environmental heat will cause women's bodies to build up heat more easily than men's bodies do. That's why women are more likely to be affected adversely by external heat. Interestingly, however, studies have shown that when women who have a predominantly sedentary lifestyle increase their level of physical activity, their bodies develop a greater tolerance to heat. So, among its many other benefits, an increase in exercise improves the body's sweating mechanism and, therefore, its ability to withstand the heat.

S*exual Differences*

As young women and men reach sexual maturity. they are acutely aware that the changes in their bodies include changes in their skin and hair and are often accompanied by new skin problems. However, women have good reason to be more conscious than men are of the intimate connections between their skin and their sexual characteristics and functions. With each menstrual cycle, with pregnancy (and with contraception), with breastfeeding, with menopause can come reminders through the way their skin looks and feels.

The obvious differences in sexual and reproductive anatomy between women and men insure that each sex will have some distinct skin problems. Women may experience irritation under the breasts or vulvar itching. The two sexes have many skin infections in common (such as the yeast infection Candida), but in women, some infections can affect the vaginal membranes because these tissues are structurally related to skin.

Sexually transmitted diseases (STDs) often have rather different symptoms for women than they do for men. This can lead to difficulties in diagnosing and treating these diseases in women. Some STDs are invisible and painless in one sex, which unfortunately makes the silent transmission of the diseases possible between sexual partners. And the long-term consequences can be different. There is considerable evidence, for example, that in women, genital warts may be related to cancer of the cervix, whereas the relationship between this STD and cancer is much less clear for men.

Many women (but not all) notice changes in their skin at various stages of their menstrual cycle. Those changes are responses to the sex hormones that the ovaries, adrenal gland, and the pituitary (a small but extremely important gland in the brain) produce. From puberty on, the levels of the sex hormones—estrogens, progesterone, and androgens—and other kinds of hormones circulating in the blood are in a dynamic equilibrium. Changes in the level of one hormone will affect the others, as well as the functions of the body that are coordinated by the hormones and the nervous system in an elegant set of feedback loops.

The interplay of the hormones is astonishingly complex, and the more we discover about it, the more complicated it looks. For example, even though estrogens are commonly described as "female" hormones or "feminizing" sex hormones and many sexual characteristics that were considered distinctively female were ascribed to their activity, men's bodies also produce estrogens and respond to them. And vice versa: the androgens, the "male" or "masculinizing" sex hormones—including testosterone—are made by women's ovaries as well as by men's testes. The level of testosterone in women can affect, among other things, patterns of hair growth, acne, and experience of menopause.

True, women on the average have higher levels of estrogens and lower levels of androgens than men, but the relative amounts vary considerably from individual to individual and over the course of the lifetime. Moreover, the two classes of hormones are quite similar in chemical structure (they are both steroids) and the body is capable of transforming one into the other. After menopause, when the ovaries produce much less of the estrogenic hormones, the androgens in women's body fat are converted to estrogens.

During that marvelously intriguing sexual state known as pregnancy, the signals going back and forth among the hormones, the various organs of the woman's body, and the fetus get even more intricate and involve a whole new world of skin interactions. The skin over the breasts and abdomen has to stretch farther and farther over the course of nine months, and then return more or less to its original size. The color of the skin can change in disconcerting ways during pregnancy. And, because the skin can absorb chemicals from cosmetics, ointments, lotions, and other topically applied medications, a pregnant woman needs to think about what effect they might have on the fetus as well as herself.

But we know far less about all this than we'd like. In this book, when I say that a certain skin condition is the result of hormonal changes—whether normal changes or ones that need medical attention—I wish I could give more details about just how the hormones act on the skin, but most of the time no one really knows.

Sometimes it seems the effects of hormones on the skin are direct and very specific: in nursing mothers, for example, hormones stimulate glands in the skin around the nipples to swell.

At other times, the effect is more roundabout. The temporary decrease in extensibility in women's skin before menstruation that I noted earlier is a good example of the interaction between the structure of skin and hormones. If you think your skin feels tighter just before your menstrual period, you're right: at that point in the cycle, your hormones are signaling to many different kinds of cells in your body to hold on to water. Cells in an inner layer of the skin respond by retaining water; as they swell, they push on the outer skin layers, and your skin feels taut.

Another result of these signals is that your internal temperature may rise temporarily several days before menstruation begins—the luteal phase of the menstrual cycle. Your skin is holding on to water, so you sweat less; and—through a related set of hormonal directions—the blood vessels in your skin constrict. Both of these physiological changes mean that the body preserves heat more readily and your temperature goes up slightly.

Some diseases with skin complications are much more common in women than men. Patients, physicians, and researchers can't help but suspect a hormonal link when they see that the illness first strikes at puberty or that the symptoms flare up in phase with menstrual cycles or change during pregnancy. The autoimmune disease called systemic lupus erythematosus (SLE or lupus, for short)—which strikes women ten times more often than men—is a notable example. The hormonal connection seems pretty obvious, but we know frustratingly little about how or why it happens.

Socially Determined Differences

Many of the differences between women and men are social rather than biological. Wherever men and women follow different fashions, wear different kinds of clothing, hold different kinds of jobs, and do different tasks at home, their skin is apt to reflect those differences.

Some of these differences create interesting but not very serious medical problems. Women who shave their legs and armpits and men who shave their faces will have similar problems with rashes and ingrown hairs, but in different places on their bodies. In cold weather, men's trousers chafe their upper legs while women wearing skirts and hosiery find their lower legs get chapped.

But differences in clothing styles can have much more important consequences: to clinch the argument that sunburns can dangerously damage the skin, researchers showed that the parts of the body most exposed to the sun by the different swimsuit designs worn by women and men were the parts most likely to have skin cancers.

Quite often the clothing you wear is determined by the kind of job you have. If you are expected to wear high heels to work, for example, you should take care to prevent ingrown toenails. When it comes to job-related skin problems, though, the differences between women and men go well beyond matters of style. In fact, it's hard to think of a line of work that does not put special stress on some part of the skin.

Women in the labor force have traditionally been concentrated in nursing, teaching, cleaning, service, clerical work, and light industry. Those jobs can expose the skin to powerful chemicals, solvents (take a look at the labels of such commonplace office items as correction fluids!), cleaning fluids, dyes, irritating materials, wounds, infections, or even just too much water. So can work in and around the house. As women move into jobs that once went chiefly to men—whether construction work or high-level management—they, and their doctors, have to be on the lookout for new kinds of skin problems that can be traced to their occupations. Whatever your work, if you are pregnant, or hoping to be, you have to consider the possibility that your skin's exposure to toxic materials on the job can harm the fetus.

Then there are the rather considerable gender-based differences in social pressures about physical appearance and attractiveness. Many of these involve the skin—especially the quality of facial skin—as well as the hair, nails, and body shape and size.

In my practice as a dermatologist, I have heard from both men and women that the way other people judge their skin's health and appearance has a real impact on their social acceptance, sexual appeal, and job opportunities. But few would deny that the women feel the stronger pressure to look attractive. The rise in cases of anorexia nervosa and bulimia (both of which can hurt the skin) among women has to be ascribed in part to their perception that society requires them, as women, to conform to certain standards of beauty.

Although definitions of beauty vary from group to group, good looks are often measured in terms of an idealized notion of youth. In great numbers, women (even young ones) turn to a wide array of commercial skin care products, cosmetics, and medical and surgical interventions, like anti-wrinkle creams, chemical face peels, dermabrasion, liposuction, varicose vein injections, and face lifts that offer the hope of a more youthful looking skin. While these products and procedures are not exclusively the domain of women, it is women who use them with far greater frequency and have the most to lose if they are not safe and effective.

A very welcome development in recent years is the new alertness, on the part of women and their doctors, to the ways women's health—and health care—can be affected by biologically and socially determined differences between the sexes. There is still a tremendous amount to be discovered, though. In the meantime, you and your doctor should work together to make sure that these factors are taken fully into account in your own case. I hope that this book helps.

Chapter 2

Basics
. . . .

Why We Have Skin
. . . .

When people think of the organs of the body, the skin is usually not on that list. But, not only is it an organ, it's our largest one, making up 15 percent of the body's total weight. Were it to be stretched out like a sheet, it would measure about two square yards.

Like the body's other organs, the skin is dynamic and essential to life, and its functions are remarkably varied. The first—and so obvious that it's easy to forget—is protecting our inner organs. Or, as a dermatology professor put it in one of his lectures: "You've got to have skin to keep your insides in!" The skin prevents damage to internal organs both from visible agents, such as clothing, plants, and chemicals, and from invisible agents, such as ultraviolet light and microorganisms.

> The skin, our largest organ, makes up 15 percent of the body's total weight.

The skin is a metabolic center, actively participating in the synthesis of many of the body's basic constituents. Carbohydrates, proteins, lipids, and amino acids are all manufactured to some degree in the skin. Also, vitamin D_3, an essential ingredient in bone formation, is metabolized in the skin. Blood vessels running into the skin carry these nutrients in and out of the skin to the rest of the body.

The skin also moves materials from outside the body to the inside. It has the ability to absorb a certain percentage of what is applied to it. Most inert products, such as water and bland creams, just stay in the skin. However, some chemicals or drugs can be absorbed to a significant degree when applied to large areas on the skin. Nowadays, certain drugs, like estrogen, scopolamine, and nicotine, are delivered to the body via a small patch applied to the skin, thereby "cashing in" on the ability of the skin to absorb.

The skin is the body's largest sense organ, responding to touch and to temperature through specialized cells. The temperature-sensitive cells—called *thermoreceptors*—react to heat by stimulating sweating, which releases body heat. In response to cold they can induce shivering to generate body heat. The thermoreceptors are closely linked to the control of blood vessels in and below the skin. So, in warm weather, the blood flows freely and the skin has a red tinge and feels warm. In cold weather, the blood vessels contract, imparting a bluish tinge to the fingers and toes.

Specialized touch receptors (known as *Meissner's corpuscles*) are located all over the skin. They are more numerous in the sensitive parts of the body, namely the fingertips, lips, underarms, and genitalia. Heat, cold, anesthetics, and other factors can dull these receptors.

Layers of the Skin

Although the term *epidermis* is frequently used as a synonym for the *skin*, it is actually the name for the outermost layer only. Two layers of skin lie beneath it—the *dermis* and the *subcutaneous tissue*.

The Epidermis

The outermost layer—the epidermis—varies in thickness from less than .1 millimeter on the genitalia to about 1.5 millimeters on the heel of the foot. The epidermis itself is made up of four layers—the stratum corneum, the stratum granulosum, the squamous cell layer, and the basal cell layer—each of which performs an important function.

The *stratum corneum*, or *horny layer*, is the outer coating of the epidermis. It consists of compacted dead cells called *keratin*, a dried-out protein. This is the layer of the skin that we feel and see. It can be smooth, soft, oily, flaky (as in dry skin), or quite thickened (as in psoriasis).

Right beneath the stratum corneum lies the *stratum granulo-*

sum, or the *granular layer*. It functions as the feeder of dead or dried out keratinocytes (skin cells) to the stratum corneum.

Next is the *squamous cell layer*, and the cells that make it up are the most abundant cells of the skin. They function as a transport medium for water. Squamous cells are, therefore, well suited to serve that same purpose for topically applied medications. Most blisters, whether from friction or from the blistering diseases—for example, herpes simplex (cold sores or genital herpes)—form within the squamous cell layer. The squamous cells produce the keratin for the outermost layer, the stratum corneum.

The *basal cell layer*—the lowest layer of the epidermis—produces the squamous cells and houses the *melanocytes*. Melanocytes are cells that make melanin, the skin pigment. Everyone has more or less the same number of melanocytes. The differences in skin color from person to person or between and among ethnic groups or races are due to differences in the *activity* of the melanocytes. These cells put forth more melanin, on the average, in Blacks than in Asians or Latinos, and a good deal more than in Whites. Since melanin protects the skin from sun damage, the darker your *natural* skin color is, the more resistant it is to damage from the sun. (Skin darkened by sun exposure does not count: it does not provide more protection for sun damage.) But even if you have dark skin, and no matter what your race is, it is still best to use sunscreen.

> The darker the natural color of the skin, the more resistant it is to damage from the sun.

There are several skin diseases and conditions that are related to the melanocyte function. Among these are malignant melanoma, albinism, vitiligo, and postinflammatory hyperpigmentation (see chapter 8).

Cells of the basal cell layer take about two weeks to migrate upwards to the stratum corneum. There they are compacted and, after another two weeks, they are shed. Thus, the usual turnover time of the epidermis—the time it takes for cells to migrate from the basal cell layer to the point of being shed from the stratum corneum—is about one month.

The Dermis

The second layer of the skin, the dermis, varies in thickness from one to four millimeters. It is thickest on the back of the body and thinnest on the palm of the hand. The dermis is made up of three different types of skin fibers: *collagen, reticulum,* and *elastin.*

Collagen is the backbone of the dermis, making up 70 percent of its weight and providing most of its strength. Wrinkles form in the skin when collagen sags. Reticulum fibers help link bundles of collagen together, while elastin fibers help the dermis remain pliable.

> **Wrinkles form when collagen—the backbone of the dermis—sags.**

Nerves, blood vessels, and lymph channels course through the dermis. The dermis is a storage place for a significant portion of the body's water. When women retain water during certain phases of their menstrual cycle, the dermis often swells. That is what causes the sensation of tight skin.

The Subcutaneous Layer

The innermost layer of the skin is the subcutaneous layer. It is composed of fat. In most areas of the skin, it is thicker than the dermis. However, it is absent in areas such as the eyelids, the nipple, the areola, and the shins. Also, the distribution of this fatty tissue is different in women than in men. Like the dermis, the subcutaneous layer contains nerves, blood vessels, and lymph channels. The main purpose of the subcutaneous layer is to serve as an insulator in order to conserve body heat. It also functions as a shock absorber to protect the internal organs against trauma.

> **The subcutaneous layer insulates the body and conserves its heat.**

The Glands

Like the rest of the human body, the skin contains glands. Basically, glands are organs that secrete a substance that regulates some aspect of the body. There are internal and external glands. Some internal glands secrete hormones. The pancreas, for example, secretes insulin, the powerful hormone that controls the body's sugar. The thyroid gland secretes thyroid hormone, which governs our metabolism. Other internal glands—such as the parotid glands in the mouth (the glands that swell up when you get mumps)—produce enzymes that help break down food.

There are three different types of skin glands: the *sebaceous* glands, or oil, glands; the *apocrine,* or scent, glands; and the *ec-*

crine, or sweat, glands. These three gland types have their roots in the dermis, but they are derived from epidermal tissue that migrates downward during the third month of fetal life. The sebaceous and the eccrine glands bring oil and sweat from the deep dermis to minute openings at the surface of the skin. But before talking about glands, a word or two about pores, which are very closely associated with the glands.

Pores

Pores are tiny openings in the skin surface. They tend to be visible on the cheeks and not very noticeable on the rest of the body. They are physically associated with the sweat and oil glands. Thus some exude oil, and others, sweat. At every hair follicle (a small body cavity or sac that a hair can grow out of) there is a pore, although not all actually have a hair growing from them. However, the pores associated with the hair follicles that have hairs growing from them are the pores that produce oil. The sweat pores are not associated with hair follicles or hair.

The Sebaceous Glands

The sebaceous, or oil, glands, are attached to hair follicles. These glands are found everywhere on the skin except the palms of the hands and the soles and tops of the feet. Sebaceous glands enlarge in response to male hormones, which are present not just in men but, in varying degrees, in women. Once the glands become functional, they continuously form oil by themselves, without any nerve stimulation. It is the increase in oil production that is one of the factors responsible for the development of acne during puberty (see chapter 3).

The Apocrine Glands

The apocrine, or scent, glands are quite active in animals. They play a prominent role during the mating season. Mammals with sensitive noses are aroused by the apocrine secretions of the opposite sex. In humans, apocrine glands are found mostly in the underarm and pubic areas. They do not become active until puberty. These glands are the only skin glands whose activity decreases during pregnancy. Therefore, certain diseases that affect them improve during pregnancy. Fox-Fordyce disease is one such example (see chapters 3 and 4).

Like the sebaceous glands, apocrine glands are attached to hair follicles. However, their distribution is much more limited than the sebaceous glands. A helpful way to remember the location of the apocrine glands is to use what I call the *a* rule: apocrine glands are found in the *a*xillae (underarms), *a*reolae (nipples), and *a*nogenital areas. These glands put forth a tiny but continuous secretion of apocrine sweat. The sole function of apocrine sweat is as a source of body odor, whereas eccrine sweat (see below) functions to regulate body temperature as well.

The total amount of apocrine secretion produced by the body is quite small. Hence, there are no untoward physical consequences from the over- or underactivity of these glands. It should also be noted that the wax-producing glands of the ear canal are modified apocrine glands. The mammary glands, also, are variations of apocrine glands.

The Eccrine Glands

The third set of glands are the eccrine, or sweat, glands. These are true sweat glands in that they regulate the body's temperature by delivering water to the skin surface so that heat can be lost by evaporation. Unlike the sebaceous and apocrine glands, eccrine glands are not associated with hair follicles.

There are two types of eccrine glands: (1) those that respond to emotional stress, such as those in the palms of the hands, and (2) those that respond to heat stress, such as the sweat glands on the rest of the body. The armpits contain both types.

When our eccrine glands work at their maximum pace, we can sweat up to 2 liters an hour!

Human sweat, though salty, is less salty than blood. When eccrine glands work at their maximum pace, the human body can sweat up to 2 liters an hour! Heat stroke and intolerance, miliaria (found commonly in infants), and drug-induced diminished sweating are all pathological conditions involving the eccrine glands.

Skin Characteristics

Thickness, toughness, stretchiness, and bounciness—these are all characteristics of the skin that allow it to carry out its essential functions. Because the skin is an external organ, these characteristics are very visible to the world and can affect your appearance.

To be able to say whether skin is tough or delicate depends on how you define and measure these terms. Do they refer to how thin or thick the skin is *or* to how easily the skin gets irritated? This is not an easy question to answer.

Measuring thickness is a fairly easy matter. One way to do this involves the use of sound waves. An interesting study was done using just this technique. One of the questions it asked was whether age affected skin thickness. A number of people of both sexes participated in the study. Their ages ranged from as young as five to the ripe old age of ninety. The results showed that skin thickness increased from age five to age fifteen and then remained constant until age sixty-five. After that, the skin became progressively thinner.

But, does thicker skin mean tougher skin? One way toughness has been defined is in terms of susceptibility to skin irritation. This has led to studies that use common chemicals—including soaps and detergents—to measure toughness. However, still more work is needed in order to determine whether thickness and toughness (or delicacy) are related.

It is also possible to measure skin extensibility—the ability of the skin to stretch. Differences in extensibility follow much the same developmental pattern as thickness does, holding steady until the seventh decade of life and then falling off. An important factor determining skin extensibility is water content: the skin needs a certain amount of water in order to stretch. The skin's ability to stretch without breaking open is critical at times of weight gain (not only in pregnancy), or in response to the stretching required by some operations and medical procedures, such as breast implants.

The skin's elasticity is related to extensibility, but different. Elasticity refers to the ability of the skin to bounce back to its original shape *after* being stretched. Unlike thickness and extensibility, both of which maintain themselves until the seventh decade, elasticity begins to decrease steadily from childhood. The elasticity of a seventy-year-old is about two-thirds that of a ten-year-old. When you were a kid, you could pinch your skin and see it bounce back to its original position. As you get older, though, the pinch is more apt to hold its shape.

The Hair

Like the glands, hair is an epidermal structure that has its root in the dermis. Hair follicles are present on all skin surfaces except the palms of the hands and the soles of the feet. Some of the hairs on the body are *vellus* hairs, which are very fine and short. Women can have quite a few vellus hairs on the face. However, most of the hairs on the body are *terminal* hairs. These vary in appearance but are longer, coarser, and far more easily visible than the vellus hairs.

The average scalp has one hundred thousand hairs. The scalp hairs are the fastest growing hairs on the body. They grow about one-third of a millimeter per day, or roughly one inch in two months. In Whites, the hair shaft is straight, producing relatively straight or wavy hair. The hair shaft in African Americans is coiled, producing coiled hair, and can be drier and more brittle than the hair of most Whites. As a result, it can be more difficult to manage.

Scalp hairs grow roughly one inch in two months.

The hairs on the scalp go through a resting, or *telogen*, phase and an active growth, or *anagen*, phase. At any given time, about 90 percent of scalp hairs will be in the active growth phase while only 10 percent will be in the resting phase. The active growth phase lasts for several weeks to months, until the new hairs grow in and replace hairs that have been lost, which is generally about seventy-five to one hundred per day. When the hair is in the anagen phase, virtually all the hairs that are normally lost in a day are replaced with new ones. During this phase the hair continues to grow out from the scalp and thus can grow longer.

Scalp hairs can remain in the growing (anagen) phase for years. But when they enter the telogen phase growth is stopped, and no hairs come in to replace the ones that are shed each day. Thus, during the telogen phase the overall number of hairs on the head decrease, and the hair doesn't grow longer.

Scalp hairs are capable of growing much longer than the hairs on the rest of the body because they go through such long anagen phases. By contrast, pubic hairs enter the anagen phase for only a few months per year, after which they return to the telogen phase. That's why these hairs stay comparatively short. The formation of hair, wherever it grows on the body, is quite similar to the formation of the stratum corneum of the epidermis (the skin's outermost layer). The cells of the hair follicle grow upward toward the center shaft. When those cells die they are compacted into the protein substance known as hair, just as the dead cells in the stratum corneum are compacted into keratin.

Warm weather stimulates hair growth; freezing temperatures stifle growth.

Warm weather stimulates hair growth; freezing temperatures stifle growth. Emotional or physical stress sometimes will cause hair to go into the resting (telogen) phase. Baldness occurs when the hairs go into a permanent telogen phase (see chapter 7).

The Nails

Nails are also epidermal structures that migrated into the dermis during fetal life. To understand how nails grow, let's take a look at how the body makes them. Under the cuticle, at the bottom of the nail, is an area known as the *matrix*. The matrix is the nail-manufacturing plant of the body. It takes cells and packs them tightly into a tough protein called keratin. Keratin, a conglomeration of dead cells, is what the nails are made of. The pink color of nails is caused by the bed of blood vessels that lies underneath them.

You may be asking yourself why so many things: the outer layer of the skin, the hair, *and* the nails, things that look and feel so different, can all be made of the same substance—keratin. The reason is that the keratin in these different structures, although similarly composed (of dried out, dead protein cells), is compacted differently in each.

Unlike the outer layer of the skin (the epidermis), the nail does not have a layer beneath it comparable to the granular layer of the skin. Instead, there is a cementing substance that keeps the nails fastened to the nail bed. If the nail gets separated from the underlying nail bed, a granular layer can form. This can make it difficult for the nail to reattach.

Some interesting trivia about nails: Nails grow at the rate of .1 millimeter a day, or roughly one-third as fast as hair grows. Do fingernails grow faster than toenails? Indeed they do. In fact, fingernails grow almost twice as fast as toenails. It takes

Nails grow at the rate of .1 millimeter a day, or roughly one-third as fast as hair grows.

a new fingernail six months to grow back, while a toenail takes about a year. Which fingernail grows the fastest? The nail of the middle finger grows faster than all the others. In right-handed people, the fingernails on the right hand tend to grow faster than those on the left. And for lefties, it is the fingernails on the left hand that grow fastest. The thumbnail grows the slowest of all the nails. The older you are, the more slowly your nails grow. And now, a final trivia question. Whose nails grow faster—a woman's or a man's? The truth is that men's nails grow faster than women's. The difference is very slight, but there is a difference. No one really knows why this is so. Nail disease may result from primary damage to the nail itself, as in direct trauma, or from contact with certain chemicals, or from fungus infections of the nail. Nail disease may also be an expression of a generalized skin disease, such as psoriasis or lichen planus (see chapter 8). But the nails also reflect what is going on elsewhere in the body, either as a result of a disease whose main target is not the skin, like thyroid disease, or from dietary irregularities, or even as a result of certain medications we may be taking.

Men's nails grow faster than women's.

Nutrition, Dieting, and the Skin

People made connections between diet and skin symptoms long before physicians knew very much about this subject. A good example is the well-known story of how British sailors noticed that when they failed to eat citrus fruit on their long voyages they developed bleeding gums and spiny skin rashes. The disease these sailors suffered, which was the result of the absence of vitamin C in their diet, came to be called scurvy. It is a skin and mucous membrane disease that begins with bleeding gums and rashes and can be fatal. To combat the problem, these seafarers would load up on lemons and limes and suck on them during the course of their journeys. (In fact, that's why British sailors are called "limeys.")

Their discovery about the importance of eating citrus fruit took place, however, long before vitamin C had been isolated or named. Eventually, medicine became more aware of the role nutrition plays in skin health and disease. Besides the connection made between vitamin C and scurvy, the inadequacy of, the total lack of, and even too much of certain nutrients—like vitamin A, niacin, riboflavin, pyridoxine (vitamin B_6), and vitamin B_{12}—have been recognized as playing a role in skin problems.

Specific Vitamins and the Skin

Lack of vitamin A produces dry eyes and skin. An overdose of vitamin A causes peeling of the skin, headaches, arthritic pains, and even liver problems. Niacin, a vitamin recently made popular for its beneficial effects upon cholesterol, can be deficient in cases of severely inadequate nutrition. This deficiency leads to pellagra, which is characterized by dermatitis, diarrhea, and dementia. The dermatitis takes the form of a sun-sensitive rash on the arms and face,

> **Insufficient vitamin A produces dry eyes and skin.**

accompanied by a V-shaped, upper chest rash referred to as "Casal's necklace." Riboflavin deficiency produces cracked lips and a groin rash. Insufficient amounts of pyridoxine (vitamin B_6) will cause a seborrheic dermatitis on the face, while a deficiency in vitamin B_{12} results in only a mild rash of the hands.

Improper Nutrition: Inadequacies and Excesses

Improper dietary intake is not the only reason for nutritional and caloric deficiencies and excesses. However, most frequently, it is the culprit. The word *malnutrition* is often thought to refer to an insufficient quantity and variety of food, mostly due to poverty and economic and social underdevelopment, and sometimes to eating disorders. However, malnutrition really refers to more than insufficient nutritional or caloric intake, and includes, for example, overeating.

Among the poor in this country, who exist in far greater numbers than many of us are aware, hunger-related malnutrition is still a problem. However, in the United States in the twentieth century, malnutrition is often related to other phenomena as well. Among these are alcoholism, dieting, obesity, and conditions like anorexia nervosa and bulimia. Some of these problems are more prevalent among the middle and upper classes, although some occur in conjunction with poverty.

Alcoholism and Nutrition

Most alcoholics eat a regular assortment of food, but many substitute alcohol for some of their meals. The result can be an invisible form of malnutrition, with implications for the ability to ward off disease. A very revealing study was conducted in 1979 at the University of Maryland School of Medicine. In cooperation with two Veterans Administration medical centers, the investigators analyzed data from 135 alcoholics. All were employed and free of any major chronic illness. When tested for signs of malnutrition, such as weight, height, mid-arm muscle circumference, and skinfold thickness of the triceps, they were found to fall within the normal range. However, when tested for their skin's ability to react to injected antigens, major differences from nonalcoholics were noted. This suggested an immunological problem.

The test itself works this way: Most adults have been exposed to germs such as Candida, the mumps virus, and strep bacteria. If antigens (proteins) of these germs are injected into the skin, there will be a localized skin reaction to fight them off. This will take the form of a red bump on the skin at the injection site. In the alcoholics studied, 40 percent had no reactions to at least two out of three of these injected antigens, whereas 100 percent of the normals reacted. This indicates that alcoholism affects the skin's reactivity to these common germs and, presumably, to many others. People suffering from forms of malnutrition also show this skin sign of a weakened immune system.

Dieting to Lose Weight

Malnutrition, in the form of inadequate caloric and nutritional intake, can result from dieting to lose weight. And although being slim can be quite reasonable for the sake of health and appearance, our culture has a major preoccupation with losing weight, with sometimes unhealthy and costly consequences for the individual. We are bombarded with direct and indirect messages to be thin. Or thinner.

One need only walk into a local bookstore to see what a prominent role dieting plays in our society. Diet books, diet guides, and anything you want you to know about dieting are there. Or, open up your local newspaper or any one of the many popular magazines that are published, and you're likely to find advertisements for dieting clubs, spas, and retreats. Turn on the TV and you'll discover which celebrity is on what diet and how much they have lost. There are physicians who specialize in weight loss. They are called bariatricians, and they offer medically supervised weight control programs. So, from popular culture to the field of medicine, dieting surrounds us. But how much is known about its effect on the skin?

A study published in the *American Journal of Clinical Nutrition* looked at changes in the epidermis during prolonged fasting. Nine persons who were markedly obese (with an average weight of 465 pounds) lost an average of seventy pounds over a two-month period. Skin biopsies before and after the two-month period revealed that the epidermis was thinned out, even though these people were still quite obese after their weight loss. This indicates that rapid weight loss can lead to thinning of the skin.

> **Rapid weight loss can lead to thinning of the skin.**

Another study, at Boston University School of Medicine, evaluated the sebaceous (oil) gland response to prolonged caloric deprivation. In eighteen obese individuals it was found that as early as five days after the restrictive diet was begun, there were alterations in the skin and the surface oils of the skin. After an average of six weeks, a 40 percent drop in sebum (oil) production was noted.

To get more insight into this subject, I contacted Dr. Martin Katahn. Many of you know him as the author of the best-selling diet books *The T-Factor Diet* and *The Rotation Diet.* He is also the director of the obesity clinic at my alma mater, Vanderbilt University Medical Center in Nashville, Tennessee. I asked if he had seen any skin effects in the people who followed his diets. Did acne get better? Did dandruff get worse? His answer to both questions was no. But he has noticed dry skin and cracked lips when people consumed less than twenty grams of fat per day. These conditions disappeared when salad dressing made with oil was substituted for the nonfat, no-oil, diet dressings his patients had been using.

Because there are certain minimum nutritional requirements for skin health and overall health, medically supervised diets are less likely to result in skin and internal complications than when diets are undertaken without qualified nutritional supervision. And, at the very least, whenever you are on a diet, it is important to let your physician know about any skin changes that you notice.

While on the subject of dieting, you've no doubt heard the popular expression that you "can't be too rich or too thin." Maybe you can't be too rich—that's a subject for another book!—but there is no doubt that you *can* be too thin. But how thin is too thin? This answer is—if you are not taking in enough nutrients to stay healthy.

There are charts that relate gender, height, and body build to what is purported to be an ideal or "normal" weight. But the weights given in these charts are based on just a few characteristics of the people they studied. In reality, the healthiest weight for each of us can be influenced by factors not considered in those studies. Thus, such charts should only be used as rough guides. Instead, each individual adult, perhaps with help from her physician, should determine what weight is best for her overall well-being.

However, social pressures regarding weight are considerable, especially on women. And, sometimes, the reaction to these pressures can be excessive, without any regard to your own health. When a person feels that *any* fat on the body is ugly or repulsive, the stage is set for the development of a potentially life-threatening disorder, anorexia nervosa.

Some eating disorders, most notably anorexia nervosa and bulimia, are seen almost exclusively in women. Typically, the disorder begins during the teenage years, in middle- to upper-class females. The sense of body proportion is distorted and every effort is made to lose weight—including crash diets, starvation, enemas, laxatives, and forced vomiting. In bulimia, these measures are often preceded by food binges. There are several skin symptoms associated with these conditions, along with numerous other consequences, including death (see chapter 8 for more on these disorders).

Obesity

Obesity creates its own set of difficulties for the skin. However, these are usually not directly related to faulty nutrition. Instead they are the result of the physical characteristics of obesity itself. Some of these same problems may occur as a result of the weight gain involved in pregnancy. Stretch marks and varicose veins are two of the more obvious ones. Sometimes in obesity overlapping folds of skin rub up against each other. This will often cause a skin irritation or rash. This condition is called *intertrigo*. The damaged skin can then become infected by bacteria. Rashes can also develop between obese fingers, and these rashes can become infected. Treatment for such problems involves airing out the affected areas and using the appropriate creams and/or antibi-

Obesity can cause stretch marks, varicose veins, and a skin irritation called intertrigo.

otics. Obesity does not, however, aggravate the rashes associated with psoriasis and eczema.

The Effect of Nutrition on the Hair and Nails

The hair and the nails, as extensions of the skin, can also be affected by your nutritional status. The hair of malnourished people grows more slowly than normal and falls out more easily. While there is no one vitamin or mineral that causes hair to grow better, lack of protein, minerals, and vitamins can retard hair growth. People with anorexia nervosa develop an increase in what is known as *lanugo hairs*. These are fine hairs that are predominant on the face but can be present on the trunk and extremities as well. It has not yet been determined why this is so.

The nails may also signal problems with the body's nutritional state. Horizontal ridges of the nails, called *Beau's lines*, are similar to rings inside a tree trunk. Beau's lines may result from irregular weight loss or virtually any bodily state of illness. Horizontal white

> Prolonged anemia can lead to the formation of spoon-shaped nails.

lines on the nails, known as *Mees' lines*, result from generalized malnutrition. These white lines disappear when proper caloric intake is restored.

Prolonged anemia from a variety of causes, including chronically heavy menstrual bleeding or chronic alcoholism, can lead to the formation of spoon-shaped nails. Soft or brittle nails can result from extreme undernourishment, such as that which occurs in anorexia nervosa. There is also a decreased rate of nail growth in response to caloric deprivation, even when reasonably adequate nutrition has been maintained.

Several conditions can cause the entire nail to become a dull yellow. Called "yellow nail syndrome," this problem has been found in markedly obese people but also in conditions such as kidney failure and AIDS.

Chapter 3

Skin and the Life Cycle
· · · · · · · · · · · · · · · · ·

Introduction
· · · · · · · · · · · · · · · ·

From the very first breath of life the human body, and therefore the skin, undergoes constant change. Normal patterns of growth, your genetic makeup, your gender, past and present illnesses, hormonal fluctuations and changes, the state of your immune system, your present and previous work, your nutritional history, the environmental exposures—all help determine the way your skin looks and functions during the different stages of your life. Although each factor by itself can influence the skin, more often they interact. For example, the extent to which your skin has been exposed to the sun, which is in part related to your age, can work in combination with your genetic makeup in the development of certain skin cancers later in life. The immune system and probably a number of occupational and environmental exposures also play an important role. Similarly, the wrinkles that develop later in life are a result of certain normal maturational changes that affect the skin, but some people develop more wrinkles than others do, and at different ages. This is an example of maturational forces working together with genetic characteristics, your total lifetime sun exposure, and probably other factors as well.

Because so many things that affect the skin play themselves out within the context of the life cycle, a look at the skin at the various stages in a woman's life can shed important light on the way it looks and functions in health and disease.

However, please do be aware that not everything essential or basic about skin can neatly fit into a developmental framework. Although it is a helpful way to understand the skin, very little about human beings can be understood completely by applying one simple model, or by using neat, clear-cut categories, or by placing information into neat little "boxes." In fact, that's what makes the study of human beings so exciting and challenging— even if at times a bit frustrating! Just as soon as you think everything fits nicely into place, up jumps an exception that just doesn't want to fit in at all.

But not to worry! Let me give you the interesting exceptions and qualifications to the life cycle approach right here, at the outset, before you get started, in order to place the material in this chapter in its proper perspective.

1 ▶ Since many skin conditions and diseases are not age specific, they will not be discussed here but will appear later, in chapter 8, which is devoted exclusively to skin diseases and conditions. However, those that are specific to pregnancy will appear in chapter 4.

2 ▶ Certain conditions can emerge at several points in the life cycle. (Acne, for example, occurs most frequently in adolescence but can also occur at other stages.) When the characteristics and consequences of conditions like these are the same no matter when they occur, I will generally discuss them with the stage of life in which they usually first occur *or* at the stage they occur with the greatest frequency. But I will also make mention of them at the other points in the life cycle, especially when they manifest themselves differently at different ages.

3 ▶ Some skin conditions—like the skin cancers—will only be mentioned briefly in this chapter, but discussed in detail in chapter 8. That way, the discussion here, of normal maturation and of age- and gender-specific conditions and diseases, won't be overwhelmed or obscured by the details of very complex, serious, and diseases that may sound a bit frightening.

4 ▶ Despite the fact that I felt that the characteristics, problems, and care of women's skin were sufficiently unique to warrant a separate book, the life cycle pattern of women's skin is not *completely* unique. In fact, I'll bet some of you have already been thinking to yourselves something like: "This is supposed to be a book about women's skin, but men get acne too." And, of course, you're right. But, much of the material *is* decidedly gender-specific to women, as you will see as you read on.

Well, if you didn't believe me before, I think you'll agree now. When it comes to human beings, little is clear-cut or simple, no matter how hard you try to make it so!

A Recommendation

I know it might be tempting to read only the section of this chapter that is devoted to the stage of life you are in currently. But if you do, here's what you may miss—

▶ some conditions that are most typically found (and thus discussed) at a stage other than your current one

▶ information that could be useful to a close relative or friend in a different age group

▶ information that might make sense of some perplexing skin problem you experienced in the past

▶ information that might help you take some useful preventive steps to minimize future problems with your skin.

Infants and Toddlers

Birthmarks

Newborn skin is soft and somewhat wrinkled. Birthmarks are common. Bluish-brown patches on the lower back and/or the thigh are known as *Mongolian spots*. They are found most often in the babies of African Americans, but some Asian babies and some White babies have them also. There is no medical significance to these spots and most resolve with time. The case is very different with raised brown birthmarks. These never disappear.

A general rule of thumb concerning birthmarks is that the

| All congenital moles should be regularly checked for changes by a physician. |

larger they are, the more potential for them to become malignant later in life. Very large, hair-bearing birthmarks, called *bathing trunk nevi*, have a high rate of transformation into malignant melanomas. *All* congenital moles should be regularly checked for changes by a physician. This is especially important after puberty. In fact, many physicians recommend having them removed *before* there is any sign of malignancy, as a preventive measure. (For a more complete discussion of this issue, see the section called "The Sixties and Up" later in this chapter. See also chapter 4.)

Flat, red birthmarks, called *portwine stains,* can occur anywhere on the body but are more common on the head and neck. These are not dangerous but may be quite disfiguring. Recent advances in laser surgery make it possible for portwine stains to be removed without leaving scars (see chapter 6).

Sun Exposure

With the ever-diminishing ozone layer, it is vital to begin sun protection at an early age. It is estimated that 80 percent of a person's lifetime sun damage occurs *before* the age of twenty. According to a Harvard University study, it only takes one severe sunburn before the age of eighteen to double your risk of developing malignant melanoma.

The fairer the skin, the higher the risk. Thus, extra special care should be exerted with White children who have blonde or red hair. Sunscreens should be used with *all* children, however, and protective clothing should be worn. Hats are very important, since 85 percent of all skin cancers occur in the head and neck region. Make a point of carrying SPF 15 (or higher) sunscreen with you. ("SPF" stands for "sun protection factor," which is explained in more detail in chapter 5.) Spread it on the baby's or child's skin. If they are old enough, teach them how to apply it themselves, but supervise them. We really can't expect kids to understand the importance of this "unfun" task. However, as you probably know, sun exposure must be monitored and protected against throughout life, not just in young children. So don't just carry and use sunscreen for the kids. People of all ages should use it whenever they are exposed to the sun.

> All children—no matter what their skin color—should use sunscreen, hats, and clothing to protect against sun damage.

The Skin as a Telltale Sign of Child Abuse

Child abuse is a serious and disturbing problem in our society. The statistics are staggering. Each year more than two million children are abused and more than four thousand die from abusive treatment. It is the leading cause of death in children aged six to twelve months.

According to Dr. Lawrence Schachner of the University of Miami Department of Dermatology, child abuse victims tend to be those children who are the most helpless. Two-thirds are under three years of age, and handicapped children are the second largest group.

Often the first, and sometimes the only, noticeable sign of abuse is on the child's skin. Ninety percent of all abused children will have some indication of that abuse on their skin. If we, as adults, are to be responsible about the problem of child abuse in our society, we need to know how to detect the possibility that child abuse has taken place. To do so, we must acquaint ourselves with its skin manifestations and how best to deal with that knowledge.

> **Ninety percent of all abused children will have some indication of that abuse on their skin.**

Bruises are the most common skin signs of child abuse. They differ in several ways from the bruises children usually receive in the ordinary course of play. When kids fall while playing they tend to injure areas of bony prominences, such as their elbows, knees, forehead, or the chin. Bruises caused by abuse are more likely to be on the child's cheeks, thighs, or buttocks. Another clue to an abusive bruise is that it will sometimes assume the shape of the instrument of that abuse. Hence the bruise can have the appearance of a handprint, the curve of a fingernail, tooth marks, or the outline of a belt buckle.

Another common skin sign of abuse is a burn. The two main types of abusive burns are contact burns and scalding burns. A contact burn can also reflect the instrument of abuse. For example, it might look like (and be) a cigarette burn. An abusive scalding burn, which results from someone deliberately holding the child's skin in a hot liquid, usually has distinct borders. This differs from a scalding burn from a hot liquid that splashed onto the child's body. Such burns tend to be accidental rather than intentional, and usually vary in size, shape, and depth.

But these guidelines to the differences between the skin bruises and burns that result from accidents or play and those that result from abuse are not absolute or written in stone. The diagnosis of child abuse requires considerable experience and skill. Ultimately, it is a diagnosis that is best made by people who are expert in dealing with this problem.

The more difficult-to-detect form of child abuse is sexual abuse. The visible skin signs of this kind of abuse are on the anal and genital areas of the body—areas that are usually only seen by those who are involved in the direct and close care of the infant or young child.

The skin manifestations of some of the viral sexually transmitted diseases (see chapter 8) are warts, herpes simplex eruptions, and molluscum contagiosum. But, because warts are so common in kids, if they appear in the anal or genital areas you might be tempted to dismiss the possibility that they are evidence of sexual abuse. However, warts do not commonly occur in the anal or genital areas of the body unless they are the result of sexual contact. And this is especially true if the child shows no evidence of warts elsewhere on the body.

Childhood

Contagious Skin Diseases

As children develop physically and mentally, they move out into the world, often far more rapidly than their weary parents or caretakers would like! This widening experience with new activities, people, and environments is very important to their healthy development, but it does expose them to a whole new range of germs. Adding to this is normal childlike carelessness—they simply don't appreciate the relationship between sanitation and disease. Hence, quite naturally, kids play in dirt, with open cuts on their hands, wipe those dirt-covered hands on cuts or open sores that might exist elsewhere on their body, and rub those hands on their mouth and nose. They also are exposed to other children and adults who might harbor infectious skin conditions. All this creates many possibilities for them to become infected.

There is another contributing factor. Because these are often first-time exposures, young children haven't had the chance to build up immunity to these germs (infectious agents). So, it's not just that they are experiencing a wider range of germs; they haven't had a chance to develop immunity to them. That's why kids are so much more vulnerable than are healthy older children, adolescents, and adults to the very same infectious agents.

Among the common contagious skin diseases of childhood are: (1) warts, which are caused by viruses, (2) impetigo, which is caused by bacteria, and (3) certain fungal infections, like ringworm of the scalp. Let's have a closer look at these conditions.

Warts

A wart is a contagious growth caused by a virus. Almost everyone gets one at some time during their life. Warts are quite common in childhood and even more common among teenagers. In fact, it is estimated that about 10 percent of all teenagers have warts. In adulthood, their prevalence declines because as the body matures it builds up resistance to the viruses that cause warts. That is not to say that grown-ups don't have their troubles with warts. In fact, in adults, warts are often more difficult to get rid of than they are in teenagers or children.

About 10 percent of all teenagers have warts.

Since effective vaccines have been developed for other viral diseases—like polio, rubella, mumps, and measles—a good deal of thought has gone into the development of a wart vaccine. But there are difficulties with this. For not only are there many different kinds of warts, like the so-called common wart, the flat wart, and mosaic warts; there are over fifty types of wart viruses. For example, wart virus types 6, 8, and 11 cause the common "finger wart" varieties of warts, while types 16 and 18 are the ones that tend to be sexually transmitted, causing warts in the genital areas (see chapter 8). In order for vaccines to be effective, they must be capable of stimulating immunity to the particular germ—for example, the virus or bacterium—that causes the disease. Thus, an effective vaccine against warts would have to stimulate immunity to the over fifty different viruses that cause warts, and that is too tall an order given our current technology in developing vaccines.

Actually, many warts go away by themselves—the immune system can fight off warts without any outside help. Sometimes, in fact, your immunity is sufficient to prevent them from developing in the first place.

Interestingly, there is strong evidence that getting rid of warts can be psychologically induced. The reason for this is not well understood. In an effort to mobilize the psychological forces that apparently affect the immune system's ability to fight wart viruses, some people turn to techniques like hypnosis and visualization. In addition, there are many folkloric "cures" for warts, such as shaking your finger at a passing train, rubbing the wart with an old potato, or burying an old sock. And sometimes these efforts do work! It is felt that these approaches induce a psychological state that somehow enables the immune system to overcome the warts and eliminate them.

It has been noted that with multiple warts if you kill the "mother wart," the baby warts will go away. A patient came to see me who perhaps had the all-time worst case of palmar warts I have ever seen. She was a nineteen-year-old young woman who was beleaguered with scores of large warts on her palms. After talking the situation over with her at length, we decided to remove only the two largest warts on each palm so as not to totally disable both of her hands. With that done, she was to come back in two weeks to have the remaining warts—or some more of them—removed. Upon her return, incredibly, all of the rest of her warts had disappeared! She was free of warts for the first time in years. I believe this was probably due to an immunological response induced by the departure of the mother warts. This experience underscores the need for medical research into how folk techniques work—research that has already produced some important drugs and methods now being used in modern medicine.

Folkloric techniques, however, are by no means ones you can bank on to rid yourself of warts. Even medical interventions are sometimes unsuccessful. Quite often, warts are very resilient and can persist for years. Depending on where they are or how many there are, they can be a cosmetic problem and, thus, embarrassing. Many warts are painful, especially those on the sole of the foot. And, of course, warts are contagious. They can spread to other people through direct contact or to another site on the body of the person who already has them.

There are various methods of removing warts. Some are slower, some are faster, and some are more effective at preventing the more resilient warts from growing back. A method that has been around for a long while involves the frequent application, by the physician and/or the wart sufferer, of topical acids. The acid slowly eats away at the wart virus. That, in combination with the frequent paring down of the surrounding callus, is often successful.

Not everyone is patient enough to go through the acid removal procedure and to wait and see if the acid will work to remove the wart. And, for certain warts, a more aggressive approach is needed. In such cases liquid nitrogen freezing can be used. Liquid nitrogen is a cold compressed gas that is stored at $-196°$ C. When sprayed or applied to a wart, it freezes the virus and kills it. Its drawbacks are that it can be uncomfortable to downright painful, and multiple sessions are still generally necessary because not all of the viral load is killed by a single freeze. Liquid nitrogen therapy is often combined with home acid treatments for a one-two punch.

A still quicker method involves burning off the wart. This is accomplished by first injecting a local anesthetic and then using a burning needle, known as a hyfrecator, to destroy the entire wart. One such treatment is often sufficient to remove the wart. However, it should be noted that if the wart is on the fingertip or palm the resultant scar can interfere with tactile sensation. Since normally, these are areas of heightened tactile sensation, the reduced sensation associated with scars can be quite noticeable and uncomfortable.

The most modern method for getting rid of warts involves the carbon dioxide (CO_2) laser. Here's how it works. Carbon dioxide is contained within a compartment that is attached to a hand-held instrument designed for laser surgery. The CO_2 is then energized by an electric current. This causes it to emit a pinpoint beam, which can be directed right at the target site on the skin.

The most modern method for getting rid of warts involves the carbon dioxide (CO_2) laser.

The CO_2 laser beam destroys the wart, with little or no scarring. That is one advantage this technique has over the hyfrecator. Another is that the pain that occurs after the local anesthesia wears off is often less. The reason for this is that the CO_2 laser seals nerve endings as it burns, thereby affording a prolonged state of local anesthesia. Also, lasered sites heal somewhat faster. And they offer another significant advantage—higher cure rates. In fact, CO_2 laser ablation is considered by most to be the treatment of choice for warts that resist cure (that keep growing back after being removed) or warts in difficult-to-treat areas.

Impetigo

The most common bacterial infection of the skin is impetigo. It is characterized by one or many crusted sores and can occur anywhere on the body. Impetigo is usually caused by streptococcal (strep) or staphylococcal (staph) bacteria. Epidemics can develop in schools, where children pass these germs from one to the other. Treatment with the appropriate antibiotic solves the problem, but many children get reinfected from their friends or relatives, and the cycle starts over again. Impetigo is not very common in adults.

Ringworm

Some types of fungal infections are more predominant in childhood, while other types appear more often in adults. Ringworm of the scalp is common in kids. It begins as a small, scaly patch or sometimes as a group of pus-filled blisters. The fungus can spread to other parts of the scalp and, if left untreated, can turn into a large, tender growth called a kerion. This growth can become so inflamed that a permanent bald patch can result if prompt treatment is not given.

> If left untreated, ringworm of the scalp can turn into a large, tender growth.

Infectious Diseases of Childhood with Skin Rashes

The fever and the itchy rash that accompany measles, rubella (German measles), and chickenpox have made many a child miserable for a week or two. It's easy to dismiss these as mere childhood diseases, but the fact is you should take them seriously because they sometimes have severe complications. Try to keep your kid from scratching the itchy red bumps; that can leave scars on the skin. Many parents and physicians swear by calamine lotion and oatmeal baths to help relieve the fierce itching.

Be sure to have your children immunized against measles and rubella. Usually one shot will cover both of those diseases, and mumps too. By offering protection against the diseases, immunization also helps avoid the severe complications they sometimes cause. Equally important, it reduces the chances that pregnant women will be exposed to the rubella virus, which is well known to cause severe birth defects. And, remember, children with rubella can spread the disease *before* the rash appears—before you even know that the child is infectious. In recent years, the failure of parents to get immunizations for their kids has led to epidemics of this disease among high school and college students, with some deaths. (See also chapter 4.)

> Children with rubella can spread the disease *before* the rash appears.

A vaccine for chickenpox is not yet available to the public, but vaccines for this disease are being developed and studied. The cause of chickenpox is the herpes zoster virus (also called varicella-zoster). This virus sometimes lies dormant for years after causing the disease in childhood and re-emerges in adulthood as shingles, a painful rash of the skin and underlying nerves. The virus can be spread by touching the shingles rash. Similarly, chickenpox can spread by touching its rash, but it is usually transmitted when the virus is airborne. Exposure to chickenpox is therefore primarily via the respiratory route rather than being the result of contact with the skin rash, as it is with shingles. And, although they sound alike, the herpes *zoster* virus should not be confused with the herpes *simplex* viruses—one of which causes sores on the lips (often called cold sores) and one of which causes the sexually transmitted disease called herpes (see chapters 4 and 8).

Noncontagious Skin Diseases

Not all skin diseases of childhood are associated with infectious agents. But, despite that, they can create considerable discomfort and often require medical intervention.

Eczema (Atopic Dermatitis)

Eczema, or atopic dermatitis, is a well-known skin condition. It sometimes is an allergic reaction, but in some cases it is a hypersensitivity reaction—a category of reaction that is broader than allergic reactions are (and one about which medicine still has a lot to learn). Although eczema occurs at other stages of life, childhood is when it most commonly first appears. Often it is found in children who also have asthma and/or hay fever. It is an itchy, red, scaly rash that can occur anywhere on the body. However, the most likely areas to be affected are the pit of the elbow, behind the knee, and around the neck.

Many cases of childhood eczema improve with age, but in many, the condition continues through adulthood. It gets worse when the cold, dry winter weather moves in and improves during the more humid and warmer summer months.

Many cases of childhood eczema improve with age.

Antihistamines are sometimes prescribed to help combat the often extreme itching associated with eczema. However, there is a good bit of controversy over whether antihistamines really directly affect the itching. Some experts maintain that when the drugs do seem to control the itching, it is because of their tendency to cause drowsiness rather than because of their ability to specifically interfere with itching. However, the fact that the newer, nonsedating antihistamines seem to work just as well as the sedating ones lends credence to the fact that antihistamines help combat itching in ways that don't just depend on their sedating effects.

The judicious use of moisturizers can help with the extreme skin dryness and flakiness associated with eczema. Application of moisturizers after bathing locks in the moisture rather than letting it evaporate. However, moisturizers have to be chosen carefully. This is because in eczema the skin is often very sensitive and reactive, and certain ingredients in some moisturizers can cause further inflammation. Topical steroids are also used to treat eczema. They help keep inflammation to a minimum and also control itching.

There have been reports in the dermatology literature that the skin of individuals with atopic dermatitis harbors more germs, specifically staphylococcus, than does nonatopic skin. This means that people with eczema are more likely to have skin infections. The treatment is topical, and sometimes systemic, antibiotics.

Children who have itchy rashes on their face from eczema can develop dark circles under their eyes, known as "allergic shiners." These children can also have some increased wrinkling of the skin underneath the eyes. These are referred to as *Dennie's lines.*

Alopecia Areata

We think of baldness as primarily a problem of older men, but one kind that girls and boys are more likely to get than grownups is alopecia areata. This is a scalp condition in which small, round bald spots begin to appear. There can be just one spot or many. The cause of these bald spots is unknown, but it is felt that stress may play a major role. Many cases resolve spontaneously, while the rest require medical treatment such as topical steroids or steroids injected directly into the bald spots. If these measures fail, a course of oral steroids may be indicated.

Strawberry Angiomas

The name strawberry angioma comes from its bright red, bumpy appearance. Usually, they appear on the face. Some of the deeper types, known as cavernous hemangiomas, can reach alarmingly large proportions. The general rule of thumb is that 70 percent of these angiomas will go away by the age of seven and 90 percent will go away by the age of nine. For those that remain, surgical removal is the only real solution, although in recent years certain types of lasers have shown promise.

A*dolescence*

Adolescence is a time of great physical, emotional, and social change. Although some of the skin conditions of childhood are outgrown, new ones emerge. Many are the result of the considerable hormonal upheaval related to sexual maturation that takes place during this stage of life. Most of the body's skin glands become more active, and this has some major consequences for the skin. Changes are also taking place in the immune system. Although all this change protects the skin of adolescents from some of the problems of the preadolescent years, it makes it more vulnerable to new ones.

B*ody Odor*

With adolescence comes an increase in underarm odor, which babies and children don't have.

With adolescence comes an increase in eccrine (sweat) and apocrine (scent) gland activity. This results in underarm odor, which babies and children don't have.

D*andruff*

Although it is not universal with teenagers, this is the period of life that dandruff generally makes its first appearance. These fine white scales on the scalp are different from the thicker, yellow scales of cradle cap that infants develop. And, dandruff tends to be a chronic condition, while cradle cap goes away. Dandruff can be controlled with various shampoos or topical steroids applied to the scalp.

A*cne*

Acne is teenage Public Enemy Number One. It affects almost every teenager to some degree or another, and many adults as well. The primary cause of adolescent acne is the hormonal change associated with sexual development, which occurs in a major way during puberty. But since not every adolescent gets acne and not every adolescent who gets acne gets it with the same intensity, there are clearly other factors that inhibit or exacerbate its development. Heredity plays a prime role.

The central role of pubescent hormonal change in acne was well demonstrated by a practice that was at its peak between 1650 and 1750 in Europe. Some male singers were castrated before they entered puberty. This was done for the sole purpose of keeping their voices high enough so they could continue to sing the soprano and alto roles in the choral music of the time. None of these *castrati*, as they were called, developed acne because they never went through the hormonal change so characteristic of adolescence and so necessary for sexual maturation.

Occasionally, an eight- or nine-year-old girl will develop a case of acne, while not beginning to menstruate until up to two years later. This is not an exception to the relationship between acne and the hormonal changes of puberty. Instead, it indicates that puberty can sometimes come on very gradually, with the early changes being those involved in producing acne, while the later ones are necessary for full pubescent change and maturation to take place.

Most cases of acne are mild to moderate, but sometimes deep nodules and cysts appear, and these can lead to scarring. Males usually have worse acne than females. This is probably due to the higher levels of testosterone in their systems.

There are a lot of different treatments for acne. Many are drying agents. There are also prescription strength creams, gels, and lotions. These may contain benzoyl peroxide, antibiotics, or combinations of the two. Tretinoin (Retin-A) was first marketed as an acne medicine but has since gained greater fame for its effectiveness against wrinkles. But, its mode of working is the same for both uses. It acts by peeling off the unwanted cells, while it generates healthier cells to replace them. This increased skin turnover helps clear up the inflammatory acne lesions.

However, oral antibiotics are still the mainstay of acne therapy. Antibiotics act to decrease the skin bacterial count, which in turn decreases the number of inflammatory lesions. Oral tetracycline is the antibiotic most commonly used. The oral antibiotic treatment of acne is often a long-term affair, and questions have been raised about the undesirable impact of long-term antibiotic use on other aspects of health. One issue that has been raised concerns the effect on immunity to other diseases. But with millions upon millions of acne patients having used antibiotics for long periods, no evidence has been produced that indicates they have any increased susceptibility to disease. As with any treatment, side effects can occur with oral antibiotics. These include vaginal yeast infections, upset stomach, and sun sensitivity. Also, long-term antibiotic use can result in bacterial resistance, necessitating a switch in the antibiotic used.

Another drug that is prescribed for acne is 13-cis-retinoic acid, known best by its brand name, Accutane. This powerful drug, taken orally, is a synthetic vitamin A derivative that acts by an unknown mechanism to decrease oil production. This leaves the skin and mucous membranes of the nose, lips, and eyes very dry, but it also dries the acne very effectively. Deep cysts and nodules can be eliminated and smaller lesions can improve as well. The limiting factors regarding Accutane therapy are the side effects. Dryness of nose and lips can lead to nosebleeds and fissures. Hair loss, blurred vision, headaches, and bone pains are less common side effects but not unheard of. Blood tests may demonstrate liver abnormalities and marked elevations of serum lipids and cholesterol.

The side effect of greatest concern to women, however, is Accutane's potential for causing birth defects. Its manufacturer thought this problem had been made clear when the drug first came out in 1981. However, several lawsuits later, the Food and Drug Administration (FDA) came within a hair's breadth of yanking Accutane from the market. The company now provides strict warnings about this potential side effect by warning women of child-bearing age of the importance of not getting pregnant while using this drug. Some women, quite naturally, worried what might happen to their babies if they got pregnant after they had stopped Accutane. Would the effect of the drug linger on even after its use had been discontinued? The manufacturer tried to address these fears in a report published in the *Journal of the American Academy of Dermatology*. This study observed several hundred women who had gotten pregnant after they had ceased taking Accutane. The report claimed that there was no increase in fetal abnormalities in these women. In assessing these results, however, one must adopt a healthy skepticism, since this study was conducted by the drug manufacturer and not by an independent research team.

The treatment of acne is not limited to oral and topical medicines. Certain physical techniques are also used and found to be quite helpful. Acne surgery—the careful extraction of whiteheads, blackheads, and pustules—helps to clear the pores and prevent formation of deeper lesions. Cold quartz lamps offer gentle heat, which helps to peel off fine layers of the impacted keratin in the pores. A light spraying with liquid nitrogen accomplishes the same thing. The technique of acne peels is a bit more involved. It removes more layers of keratin and the upper epidermis. But its deeper effects lead to better and longer-lasting results. Finally, intralesional injections of steroids—injections right into the nodules and cysts—can be used to quiet them down.

It is not always easy to know which treatment will work best for any particular patient. As with a great deal in medicine, individual differences between patients require a certain amount of judgment and experimentation. Nevertheless, this overview lets you know what is available so that you can inquire whether certain approaches that haven't already been used in your case might be worth a try.

The Twenties

This is the first full decade of true adulthood. Although some women start having children earlier and some wait until later, this is the decade when most women who bear children begin their childbearing and when they have most of their children. But, no matter when pregnancy occurs in a woman's life, it makes major demands on a woman's skin, and its effects may be long-lasting or even permanent. Because of this and because of the special skin care needs and skin conditions of pregnancy, a separate chapter— chapter 4—is devoted to this topic.

Fungal Conditions

Just as the earlier life stages had their own fungal skin conditions, so does this one. Among them are tinea versicolor and tinea pedis (athlete's foot).

Tinea versicolor (so named from the variety of colors that it can assume) is characterized by fluffy patches of red, orange, tan, or

> Multicolored patches of fungus on the body can be treated with antifungal shampoo, creams, or oral medications.

white, which appear on the trunk. A variety of treatments is available. Antifungal shampoo can be applied daily to the affected areas. To be effective it must be left on for fifteen minutes, then washed off. A week's worth of this treatment should offer a cure. For those who prefer not to stand around for fifteen minutes with shampoo on their body, a twice daily application of antifungal cream will often suffice. The most convenient method is the use of oral antifungal medication. This can offer relief in just a few days. The risk of side effects, however, increases with oral antifungal medication, even though they don't occur frequently. But, no matter what treatment approach is used, this infection may recur, especially during the spring and fall. And, of all the fungal infections, it is the least infectious.

Tinea pedis (also called "athlete's foot") is a fungal condition that occurs in adults with a much higher frequency than it does in children. This nagging, chronic condition usually is characterized by scaliness on the soles of the feet and/or itchy rashes between the toes. The toenails often become infected and can become thickened and yellow in appearance. However,

> Try to get athlete's foot infections under control before they affect the toenails.

treating the toenails presents a considerable challenge. Creams have difficulty penetrating, due to the thickness of fungus-infected toenails. Thus, when the nails are affected, oral antifungal therapy is usually required for up to one year. The CO_2 laser can help to thin down the nail, making it less painful and more easily treated. In severe cases, painful toenails may have to be completely removed. Otherwise, the treatment of this condition is reasonably simple. Common over-the-counter remedies for athlete's foot are often effective. Several of them were prescription-only drugs until recently.

Pityriasis rosea

Pityriasis rosea is a relatively common disorder in which a large oval red patch, known as a "herald patch," appears on the trunk or limbs. This is followed by a "shower" of smaller red oval patches on the trunk or face. Pityriasis rosea can last for up to two months, but then it disappears. In contrast to tinea versicolor, it almost never comes back. This condition has medical science baffled. The fact that it is essentially a one-time affliction has lead some to hypothesize that it is caused by a virus, and after it runs its course, lifelong immunity follows. Yet pityriasis rosea has never been shown to be contagious, which casts doubt upon its viral etiology. Microscopic analysis of biopsy specimens has not revealed any viral particles, further undercutting the viral argument. Thus, the cause and prevention of this condition awaits discovery.

M*oles*

Moles—the result of the appearance of nevus cells in the skin—are most often brown, but can be black or colorless. They are usually slightly raised, but can be flat as well. During your twenties, moles tend to enlarge both in number and size. The average person has about thirty moles, so it is often difficult to notice if a mole is growing at a faster rate than it was before, or faster than the other moles on your body. Although change in a mole's size, shape, or color can be a warning sign of a transformation into a skin cancer, it must be remembered that most moles that change are not cancerous.

> **The average person has about thirty moles.**

In recent years, a new mole entity, known as the *dysplastic nevus*, has been recognized and defined. Clinically, a dysplastic nevus is a mole that shows some changes in size, shape, or color, but not enough to look frankly cancerous. Microscopically, the cells of dysplastic nevi back up this observation. They appear to be in a state of transformation but are not yet cancerous. Dysplastic nevi are more common in people who have an abundance of moles. They also can run in families. The best treatment for a dysplastic nevus is early recognition and adequate excision.

A*cne, again!*

Most cases of adolescent acne begin to wane during the years of the twenties, although with many people, it continues well into your twenties and sometimes beyond. Generally, though not always, it is the most severe cases that last the longest. Early and effective treatment can be helpful in this respect, but if acne does continue into your twenties, the treatments are the same as they were for adolescent acne.

> **Postadolescent acne tends to occur in hard-working professional women in their twenties and their thirties.**

But in addition to those cases that persist from adolescence, acne can appear in women in their twenties who never had it as teenagers. Dr. Albert Kligman, the discoverer of Retin-A, calls this condition "postadolescent acne." It tends to occur with greatest frequency in hard-working professional women in their twenties and their thirties and forties as well. It is a low-grade, persistent acne, in which whiteheads predominate, accompanied by a sprinkling of pustules. Premenstrual flares are typical.

It is not known why some women develop new cases of acne in their twenties who never had it before. One theory has it that chronic stress, which leads to enhanced secretion of adrenal gland androgens (a type of hormone), might make the skin secrete more oil than usual. That causes the pores to plug up, which can result in acne.

But, as with most conditions that are attributed to stress, people (patients and physicians alike) sometimes dismiss other possible causes only later to have it discovered that the cause is biological. Nevertheless, reducing stress is generally a wise thing to do. It can be helpful both in the prevention and in the treatment of many conditions and diseases, whether or not the primary cause is stress or something biological. Another thing to bear in mind is that many people experience considerable stress and don't develop acne in their twenties. So, if stress *is* involved, it is not the whole story.

Birth control pills with a high estrogen content may improve acne; but those with low estrogen content tend to worsen acne. Birth control pills can affect the skin in other ways, too. They may bring on a condition known as melasma, the "mask of pregnancy" characterized by brown patches on the cheeks and forehead (see chapter 4). The melasma may linger for months or years after the birth control pills are stopped. If birth control pills are given post partum (after the birth of a baby), some pregnancy-related diseases may flare up.

The Thirties

The well-known "thirtysomething" crowd is in somewhat of a middle ground between younger and older insofar as the skin is concerned. This is the time of life when the undesirable effects of the sun on the skin begin to appear. The sun damages the skin's elastic tissue. This damage can be seen under the microscope and can give a pretty good idea how much exposure to the sun the skin has already had.

Wrinkles

Although most people don't develop noticeable wrinkles while they are in their thirties, wrinkles can appear during this decade, especially in fair-skinned individuals. The areas around the eyes are the usual places, but fine lines may occur on the cheeks and around the mouth as well. Wrinkles are the result of a breakdown in the elastic tissue of the skin, usually from the sun. Other factors, such as wind and certain chemicals or exposure to other modes of ultraviolet light, can also contribute to their development. (See chapter 6 for treatments for wrinkles.)

Actinic Keratosis

Along with early wrinkling come other changes associated with prolonged sun exposure. Actinic keratoses are early sun damage spots. They are red, scaly, flat or raised bumps. When left alone for several months to years they can actually progress into a form of skin cancer known as squamous cell carcinoma

Red, scaly bumps, called actinic keratoses, are early sun damage spots.

(see chapter 8). Although actinic keratoses occur more often after age sixty, in fair-skinned people or those whose work or play takes them outdoors a lot, they can appear earlier. So, no matter what age you are, if you see a red, scaly spot that does not go away, get your local dermatologist to check it out. (For a more detailed discussion of this condition see the section called "The Sixties and Up," later in this chapter.)

Seborrheic Keratosis

In this condition, just as with actinic keratosis, there are scaly bumps, but seborrheic keratoses are brown or faded in color instead of red. Some have a wart-like appearance, with a thick, cobblestone character. Others can look like actinic keratoses (raised or flat bumps), but seborrheic keratoses are never cancerous or precancerous. Despite that, it can sometimes be tricky to differentiate them from skin cancers such as a basal cell carcinoma or malignant melanoma.

Skin Cancer Awareness

It really pays to check everywhere for skin cancer. A thirty-four-year-old woman once saw me on a routine office visit for poison ivy. On her way out she said, "Oh, by the way, I have this little bump behind my ear. Could you look at it?" The little bump was hidden in a crack of skin behind her right earlobe. It looked like it didn't belong there. A biopsy showed it to be squamous cell carcinoma. Her years at the beach had finally caught up with her. Upon further examination, it was discovered that the skin cancer had spread to the parotid gland in her neck. It is likely that the reason the cancer proliferated was because it had gone undetected for such a long time. After some extensive surgery, the entire tumor was removed. Five years later she appears to be free of any recurrence. (See chapter 8 for a full discussion of skin cancers.)

Some Good News on Acne

The good news for those in their thirties is that acne usually disappears and does not return. However, for some who never outgrow their acne, there will be continued ups and downs. The prevalence of acne in the forty-year-old group is about the same as in the fifty- and the sixty-year-old group. Then, for those who are seventy and up, the rate dramatically drops off.

The Forties

During this decade of life the skin exhibits an accentuation of the processes that began in the previous decade. The effects of total lifetime sun exposure become increasingly apparent. Even if you haven't done anything earlier in your life to protect your skin from the sun, starting to do so in your forties is not too late; it will at least help prevent skin damage from further sun exposure.

Rosacea

Although there is a decreased incidence of acne in the forty-year-old group, a different acne-like process can cause problems during this period of life. It is called rosacea, and it can occur in later years as well. Rosacea begins with several pustules on the face, around the nose area. It can also spread to the cheeks and forehead. In addition to bumps filled with pus, there is a marked tendency towards redness and rather enlarged blood vessels, especially on the nose. The nose may actually swell and become beet red. Women with rosacea often have to contend with a widespread myth that rosacea is an indication that they are alcoholics, since excessive alcohol use can also cause the nose to become red in people who don't have rosacea. So, although it is true that drinking lots of coffee or alcoholic beverages can make rosacea worse, the reality is that alcohol does not cause rosacea.

> Drinking alcoholic beverages or coffee does not cause rosacea, but can make it worse.

Rosacea can continue off and on for many years. Although it generally doesn't cover as much of the face and body as acne sometimes does, it may be disfiguring if left untreated. The problem is that it's not always easy to treat. As in the case of regular acne, oral antibiotics, such as tetracycline, will often suppress outbreaks. In fact, a number of my patients have been taking tetracycline once a day for thirty years! They all maintain that as soon as they stop their single daily dose the rosacea flares up again. Recently, a topical form of metronidazole has been found to be useful in the treatment of rosacea. Metronidazole is a synthetic antibacterial compound that is used with a variety of infectious conditions. By fighting off local bacteria, topical metronidazole helps to improve rosacea. However, keep in mind that neither pills nor creams will help the enlarged blood vessels that accompany rosacea. These are called telangiectasia and are treated by either very light burning with an electric needle or by the dye laser. The dye laser method (see chapter 6) usually has a very good cosmetic effect. The common facial telangiectasia that are not associated with rosacea are treated similarly.

Sebaceous Hyperplasia

Small yellowish bumps may appear on the cheeks, forehead, and nose. This condition is called sebaceous hyperplasia. It is the result of an overgrowth of the oil glands underneath the skin. Even to the medically trained eye, the bumps may look very much like small skin cancers. Thus, doing a skin biopsy may be the only way to make the correct diagnosis. Although sebaceous hyperplasia is caused by oil gland overgrowth, the bumps do not produce oil and, therefore, do not cause oily skin.

Sebaceous hyperplasia tends to be located in visibly prominent areas and has considerable impact on appearance. That's why any technique for the removal of these lesions should attempt to keep scarring to a minimum. The CO_2 laser can offer pinpoint accuracy by destroying a minimum of tissue with maximum results. The result is usually a flat, faded spot in place of the prominent yellow bumps of sebaceous hyperplasia.

Disseminated Superficial Actinic Parakeratosis (DSAP)

An unusual skin condition (with a very long name) can appear for the first time during this decade of life. Disseminated superficial actinic parakeratosis (DSAP, for short) is made up of several rings of ridged skin. Just one or hundreds of circular ridges may form on the legs or arms. There is some question as to whether or not these progress into skin cancer. To date, there is no treatment that is 100 percent effective, although many different types have been tried.

Chondrodermatitis Nodularis Helicus (CNCH)

Another skin problem that has a long name and can make its appearance during your forties is called chondrodermatitis nodularis helicus (CNCH). It involves a breakdown in the cartilage at the top of the ear. This results in a tender bump that often is very painful, especially if you rest your head on the affected ear when you sleep. CNCH never becomes cancerous, but it does tend to persist and, because of the pain, should be removed by one method or another. Liquid nitrogen freezing often suffices. Sometimes, though, excision of the skin and part of the underlying cartilage is necessary.

The Fifties

For most women and men, the fifties are marked by a gradual slowing down of the metabolism. The circulatory system works more slowly, as does the immune system, and it is harder to shed extra pounds. For women, this is also the decade when menopause usually takes place. These internal changes can sometimes have undesirable effects on the skin. On the positive side, the incidence of fungal infections does seem to plateau during the fifties.

Blood Circulation and the Skin

When the blood moves more slowly through the body, the skin is poorly supplied with blood and will tend to dry out. If circulation to the veins of the lower legs is impeded, it can cause a condition known as *stasis dermatitis.* "Stasis" means "not moving," and stasis dermatitis is the result of blood not moving upward from lower legs, depriving the skin of

> Itching may be due to sluggish circulation but can also come from liver disease or even internal cancers.

necessary nutrients. In this condition the skin turns red and dry and often will break down, leading to the formation of leg ulcers. These can be quite painful due to the rawness and exposure of the fine skin nerves. Because the poor circulation that occurs at this age tends to be chronic, these ulcers are difficult to treat.

Just as when poor circulation causes edema (swelling) in the legs, the recommended treatment to help counteract the effects of that poor circulation is to elevate the legs. It helps the body get rid of the fluid that accumulates and isn't carried away by the normal process of circulation. It is a treatment based on simple mechanics related to gravity—the fact that fluids will run, if not impeded, from higher points to lower ones, and not vice versa (unless pumped). Thus, in order to be effective in getting the fluid out of the legs, they must be raised higher than the heart. Merely propping up the legs while you are sitting doesn't usually achieve that effect. Support stockings will also aid in decreasing leg edema.

The slowing of circulation not only affects the legs, but other parts of the body as well. One result is a general tendency to drier skin. Sometimes, localized areas of *xerotic eczema*—dry, red patches of cracked, open skin—appear. Moisturizers and topical steroids are beneficial for this problem. The adverse effect on skin nutrition caused by sluggish circulation can also result in pruritus (itching). But be aware that itching may be due to a number of other causes as well, such as liver disease or even internal cancers. It is, therefore, always important to investigate the possible causes of unexplained and uncontrollable itching and not just attribute it to a sign of aging and its related circulatory changes.

Cherry Angiomas

The trunk can become dotted with small, red bumps known as cherry angiomas. There may be hundreds of them in varying sizes, but they are quite benign and never become cancerous. A light desiccation with the electric hyfrecator can remove most of these, usually without scar formation. Anesthesia is not generally necessary for this procedure.

Purpura

Starting at this stage of life, there is an increased fragility of the blood vessels of the skin. They may break in response to minor trauma, leaving reddish-purple spots known as purpura. These usually occur on the forearms. A history of excessive sun exposure makes people more susceptible to their formation. Once someone has a tendency to develop purpura, it becomes difficult to reverse the process.

> **Reddish-purple spots called purpura occur most often on the forearm.**

Postmenopausal Acne

Postmenopausal acne originates at (or after) menopause in darker-skinned women who have large pores and a history of oily skin. Most of these women did not experience adolescent acne. As with postadolescent acne, there tend to be recurrent whiteheads and pustules. Women who have this condition may also have excessive hair on the chin and upper lip.

The probable mechanism of postmenopausal acne is this: When the ovaries cease to produce the standard female hormones, the masculinizing adrenal hormones, which were present before menopause as well, become *relatively* more dominant because of the decrease in the standard female hormones that are produced. It is a matter of ratios. In menopause, the masculinizing hormones do not increase, but the female hormones decrease (although they still predominate over the male hormones).

It is not surprising that menopause can also precipitate a case of acne, since it is hormonal change that is implicated in adolescent acne. But why only *some* adolescents and *some* postmenopausal women develop acne while others don't suggests that although fluctuating hormones might set the stage for the development of acne, other factors are involved (although they are not yet fully understood). The treatment of postmenopausal acne consists in using the same simple topical acne medications that are used during adolescence.

Flushing

Flushing during menopause is caused by a decrease in the hormone estradiol. This estrogen derivative affects the ease with which blood flows through blood vessels. When the amount of this hormone goes down, the blood vessels transport blood less evenly. The resulting sudden flow of blood in or out of some vessels and not others creates both the reddening of parts of the skin (flushing) and the sensation of warmth (hot flashes) that many menopausal women experience (although women can experience one of these symptoms and not the other). Estrogen replacement therapy restores the premenopausal balance in the blood vessels, thereby reducing or eliminating these two symptoms.

A reduced intensity flushing can occur in premenopausal women as well. It happens during the last week of the cycle before the onset of menstruation. For the relief of both menopausal and premenopausal flushing, the antihypertensive drug clonidine hydrochloride has been shown to be fairly effective.

Sixty and Up

During the years of the sixties and beyond, although certain skin problems go away, new ones inevitably emerge. And, for many, the aging process takes a considerable toll on the skin.

As the elastic tissue of the skin breaks down, wrinkles become more prominent. In addition to wrinkles, the skin becomes drier and more difficult to moisturize. Fair skin assumes more of a yellowish hue.

Some of this can be explained by the decreased function of the skin glands. The sebaceous (oil) glands and the apocrine (scent) glands are less active, presumably in response to decreased circulation of sex hormones. As a result of sun damage, decreased gland activity, and general "wear and tear," the skin gradually requires more attention and more care.

Above the age of seventy, acne is very rare, presumably due to the decreased activity of the oil glands mentioned earlier. Because the immune system is somewhat slowed down with advancing age, there is a decrease in allergic reactions of the skin, such as poison ivy dermatitis. In addition, the eccrine (sweat) glands become less active and the body tends to sweat less in response to heat stimuli. This is part of the reason why elderly persons are more susceptible to heat stroke. They are unable to rid the body of heat via the sweat mechanism as effectively as younger people.

The scalp and hair are also affected by the aging process. Hair grows more slowly, and as it begins to lose its natural color, it turns gray or white. Thinning of the hair is common in both men and women. Nails grow slower and are prone to a condition referred to as *distal onycholysis*, or splitting of the tips of the nails. Nails can also tend assume a yellowish color.

There are fewer moles on the skin as time goes by. However, more skin cancers, more precancerous growths, and more benign seborrheic keratoses develop as the years go by. The effects of those sweet days in the sun—at the beach, near a pool, in a garden or backyard—are often not seen for up to thirty to forty years after the fact; hence, skin maladies caused by sun exposure really become evident after sixty. This is especially true with respect to precancerous skin changes and skin cancer itself, since it can take up to half a century for the cells of the skin to transform into a malignancy. That's why people in this age group may develop skin cancer even if at this life stage they don't spend much time exposed to the sun. (See chapter 8 for a full discussion of skin cancers.)

Even if you don't spend much time in the sun in your sixties, you can still develop skin cancer from earlier exposure.

Actinic Keratosis

Although this condition was described in the section on the thirties, it is during this decade of life when it is more likely to occur.

A fair-skinned woman in her sixties once came to see me who had a sun-induced case of actinic keratosis. She must have had a hundred of these growths, *but* she only had them on the left side of her face and left forearm. Her right forearm and the right side of the face were both spotless. Fearing that she had developed some mysterious illness, she asked my opinion. The answer was quite simple. It turned out that the woman had been a taxicab driver for the previous twenty-five years in sunny Southern California. That's twenty-five years of driving with her left forearm hanging out of the window and the left side of her face exposed to the sun.

The growths that characterize actinic keratosis can be treated by a number of different methods. Freezing with liquid nitrogen is a commonly used technique, especially when there are many growths. The frozen areas form a blister or a scab, dry up, and fall off in one to two weeks. For larger or more resistant keratoses, desiccation and curettage with the electric hyfrecator, or even laser surgery, may be indicated. Often, when they are removed, they will be sent off for biopsy to determine if they have already progressed to full-fledged skin cancer.

An alternative way of treating very superficial actinic keratoses is with a cream known generically as 5-fluoro-uracil (5-FU). (See chapter 6 for a discussion of this treatment.)

Bedsores

For the elderly bedridden person or, for that matter, for any long-term bedridden person, bedsores can be a major problem. The constant pressure upon any area of the skin can cause the cells to necrose (die). This in turn leads to a sloughing off of the dead skin, and the sore working its way deeper and deeper. Like leg ulcers, bedsores are often painful. In the elderly, because healing is generally slow, bedsores may take quite a while to get better. A very important preventive measure with people who are bedridden is to have them turned from one side to another every few hours to relieve pressure on any particular area of the body.

Bullous Pemphigoid

Another skin condition that is more common in the sixty and older population is bullous pemphigoid. It is characterized by the formation of large blisters that can occur anywhere on the body. Bullous pemphigoid used to carry a grave prognosis before the days of oral cortisone. Fortunately, this disease can now be controlled, but it still remains a big problem for the elderly, who cannot always tolerate the high doses of cortisone required for its treatment.

Kaposi's Sarcoma

Until a few years ago, Kaposi's sarcoma was seen exclusively in people sixty and up. It consists of large red bumps that can bleed and ulcerate. Kaposi's sarcoma is actually a low-grade type of skin cancer, but it has only a slight tendency to spread. Recently, this uncommon skin disease has become well known because of its occurrence in AIDS. The reason for this association is not clear, but the immunosuppressed status of AIDS patients probably causes their skin to be susceptible to this particular type of skin cancer.

Now that we've had a look at the skin in terms of the life cycle—which often was relevant to both sexes—I want to devote an entire chapter to pregnancy and the skin, a subject that is solely the province of women.

Chapter 4

The Skin in Pregnancy

D uring pregnancy a woman's body goes through a great many changes. Some involve the skin. These run the gamut from being welcome, to quite uncomfortable, to rather serious. But treatment can pose its own set of problems, because the use of medication in pregnancy is a tricky business, and special care has to be exerted in deciding when a remedy might be worse than the problem it treats. That's why even in conditions that involve considerable discomfort, if they don't cause real harm to the woman or the fetus there can be honest differences of opinion over whether to treat, when to treat, and with what. In the more serious skin problems, drug treatment is often necessary.

The problem with drug use in pregnancy is that certain drugs, considered safe or low in risk for most adults, can cause problems for the pregnant woman or the developing embryo or fetus. So, before discussing the relationship between pregnancy and women's skin, I'll first talk about the use of cosmetics and medications in pregnancy, paying special attention to the drugs that are used for skin problems.

After that, I will move on to the effect of pregnancy on the skin, hair, and nails; the effect of pregnancy on pre-existing skin conditions; and I'll close the chapter with a discussion of the skin diseases seen only in pregnancy.

Medication and Cosmetic Use in Pregnancy

The use of cosmetics and medications is a topic of considerable concern for the pregnant woman and her doctor, for, in pregnancy,

> **If you are pregnant (or think you might be), be sure to check with your doctor about the safety of any medications you have been using.**

the woman and the developing fetus must be protected from the possibility of their adverse effects. Drugs and chemicals can work differently in pregnancy, and sometimes these differences can turn a drug that is safe to use when you aren't pregnant into a harmful one when you are—harmful for you or for the developing fetus. Even topical drugs and cosmetics—because they can be absorbed into the system—must be evaluated for safety in pregnancy.

But with many drugs and in many situations, decisions about drug use are often a difficult balancing act, with the adverse effects having to be weighed against not treating a problem or condition. This dilemma over how to evaluate the safety of a drug for use in pregnancy has, quite understandably, attracted considerable attention from the medical community as well as the federal government. Here's what's involved.

Testing Drugs for Use in Pregnancy

The scientific community, quite rightly, is not free to perform research on pregnant women, even though, from a strictly scientific research point of view, that would be the best way to evaluate the safety and effectiveness of a drug for use in pregnancy. But to prevent any possible harm to the pregnant woman and/or the fetus, a strict and special limitation is placed on the testing of drugs—pregnant women *cannot* be used in such studies. As a result, conclusions about the safety and effectiveness of a drug for use during pregnancy must be based on the following kinds of information: (1) studies of the drug's effects on animals rather than on humans; (2) laboratory tests performed in vitro (outside a living organism; for example, in a test tube); and (3) follow-up studies of pregnant women who, for one reason or another, had access to the drug and took it.

While at first glance it may seem that follow-up studies of the pregnant women who use the drug would do the trick and tell us all we need to know about the effect of the drug in pregnancy, they don't. For, in order for researchers to draw sound and valid conclusions from drug use studies, certain conditions need to be met: the studies need to be done in strictly controlled situations, with the ability to perform measurements before and after the drug is used, or the studies should be done on sufficiently large groups of people who are selected scientifically—either randomly (so that there is no bias in the selection process) or where the people studied represent the groups the research results are intended to apply to (in this case, pregnant women).

To meet such standards for drug use in pregnancy, studies would need to be done on pregnant women who were chosen scientifically, and who could be evaluated *before* they take the drug as well as *during* and *after*. But the cautions and restrictions on giving drugs to pregnant women prevent this, and should. Thus, while the research that is possible to do can provide useful information about drug use in pregnancy, this research cannot meet the highest standards of good scientific methodology.

To compensate for this limitation yet maximally protect the pregnant woman and the fetus, the Food and Drug Administration (FDA) has developed a special set of standards for drug use in pregnancy. Here's how it works. Every drug that receives FDA approval for use in the general population *also* receives a rating on its safety for use in pregnant women. Each rating, or risk category, conveys the following types of information: how the decisions about the drug's safety in pregnancy were made; what level or kind of risk was found to exist; and how that risk compares to the risks involved in *not* using the drug to treat the illness for which it is intended.

The chart that follows lists the *five* FDA risk categories for drugs used in pregnancy—A, B, C, D, and X—and gives the FDA's explanations (called *interpretations*) of each. But since some of that information can get a bit technical, here's a few words of clarification: The kind of research or clinical experience on which the safety conclusions are made varies from category to category. Some of the risk categories are based on either one sort of information *or* another—for example, *either* on controlled animal studies *or* reports generated from accumulated general clinical experience (not scientific studies). For these categories the key word is *or*—they are *either* one sort of evidence *or* another. Other risk categories, however, require that *several* conditions be met. In these categories the key word is *and*. More than one type of evidence is required to meet the standards stipulated in these risk categories.

Also, be alert to two terms—*teratogenic* and *embryocidal*. They frequently appear in the interpretations of the risk categories and also regularly appear in package inserts about the safety of a drug for use in pregnancy. A teratogenic substance is one that causes abnormal fetal development, and an embryocidal substance is one that is capable of killing the embryo.

FDA Risk Categories for Drug Use in Pregnancy

Category	*Interpretation*
Category A	Controlled studies in women fail to demonstrate a risk to the fetus in the first trimester, and there is no evidence of a risk in later trimesters, and the possibility of fetal harm appears remote.
Category B	Some animal reproduction studies have not demonstrated a fetal risk, but there are no controlled studies in pregnant women. Or, some animal reproduction studies have shown an adverse effect (other than a decrease in fertility), but these were not confirmed in controlled studies in women in the first trimester and there is no evidence of a risk in later trimesters.
Category C	Studies in animals have revealed adverse effects on the fetus (teratogenic or embryocidal or other), and there are no controlled studies in women. Or studies in women and animals are not available. This category of drugs should be given only if the potential benefit justifies the potential risk to the fetus.
Category D	There is positive evidence of human fetal risk, but the benefits from use in pregnant women may be acceptable despite the risk, for example, if the drug is needed in a life-threatening situation or for a serious disease for which safer drugs cannot be used or are ineffective.

Category X	Studies in animals or human beings have demonstrated fetal abnormalities. Or there is evidence of fetal risk based on human experience or both, and the risk of the use of the drug in pregnant women clearly outweighs any possible benefit from the use of the drug. The drug is thus contraindicated: it should not be given in women who are, or who may become, pregnant.

It should be noted that these classifications are not etched in stone. Drugs are reclassified from time to time. And perhaps the most important thing to remember is that your physician's knowledge and experience with these medications is also very important in the decision about when to use a particular drug during pregnancy.

Pregnancy and Drug Metabolism

Part of the answer to the question of whether a drug—oral or topical—will do harm during pregnancy comes from understanding how pregnancy affects drug metabolism. It must be remembered that the effect a drug has on each person who takes it is not only the result of what the drug is composed of but what happens to the drug once it enters the body—the way it metabolizes.

Pregnancy, the fetus, and the placenta all have an impact on drug metabolism in pregnancy, although some of these effects are still not very well understood. It is known that drug alterations can occur as the drug is transported by the maternal blood through the fetus, although most experts feel that the effects are minimal. Placental metabolism may play a small role in changing maternal and fetal concentrations of some drugs.

Oral and Topical Medications for Skin Conditions

Let's look at the kinds of oral and topical medications that are most frequently used for skin problems, conditions, and diseases in terms of their safety for use in pregnancy. Remember that even if you used these safely before pregnancy, you should check with your doctor about continuing to use them if you become (or might already be) pregnant.

Oral Medications

 1▶ *Antibiotics*: The penicillins and their close relatives, the ceph-
alosporins, are category B drugs. These include brand names
such as Pen Vee K, Ampicillin, Amoxil, Keflex, and Velosef.
Erythromycins are category B as well. Tetracyclines are category D, contraindicated in pregnancy due to the side effect of
permanent darkening of the teeth and bones of the fetus.

 2▶ *Corticosteroids*: Prednisone, the most commonly used oral
steroid, is category B. Others, such as dexamethasone, are
category C.

 3▶ *Antihistamines*: Some over-the-counter antihistamines such
as chlorpheniramine (Chlortrimeton) and diphenhydramine
(Benadryl) are category B drugs. Most
prescription strength antihistamines are
category C. In general, all are fairly safe
for use in pregnancy.

Antihistamines are fairly safe for use in pregnancy.

 4▶ *Contraceptives and Estrogens*: These are category X and are
absolutely contraindicated for use during pregnancy.

Topical Medications

Since topically applied drugs are absorbed through the skin, they
too have to be considered for their safety for use in pregnancy.
Most prescription strength topical creams, lotions, and ointments
are category B products. Topical antibiotics, such as clindamycin
(Cleocin-T), erythromycin (T-STAT, A/T/S, Erygel), and the acne
and wrinkle treatment cream tretinoin (Retin-A), fall into this category. Topical steroids, when used in moderation, are also category B.

There is virtually no need to be worried that pregnancy will
affect the absorption of drugs and other chemicals that are applied
to the skin. For, although pregnancy does change certain aspects of
skin absorption, it does so in ways that cancel each other out, with
a net effect of virtually no change. What happens is that much of
the weight gain during pregnancy—which is due to a build-up of
water—manifests itself as an increase in blood volume and also
better hydration of the skin. This generally results in an improvement in the penetration of topically applied drugs. Balancing that
change is an increase in the blood volume, which dilutes the concentration of the drug in the blood. The result is that in pregnancy,
skin absorption of topicals is about the same as when you are not

pregnant, although if there is any difference it might be in the direction of being a little less.

Over-the-Counter Preparations and Cosmetic Products

One day, when I was delivering a lecture on the skin in pregnancy to the Obstetrics and Gynecology Department of the St. John's Medical Center in Santa Monica, California, one of the physicians there asked me the following question. "We worry about all of the prescription drugs that we apply to the skin during pregnancy, but what about over-the-counter items? Can my patients use hair dye when they're pregnant?" The same question was raised in a physician's letter to the *Journal of the American Medical Association (JAMA)* in November of 1989. He wrote that he recommends that his patients avoid hair dyes and permanents during their first trimester and, if possible, the entire pregnancy. He also advises beauticians not to work during pregnancy, due to possible chemical exposure. Was he incorrect in his recommendations, he queried?

In response, two physicians from Toronto Hospital for Sick Children reported that several animal studies showed no toxicity and no effect on fetal development after applications of twelve different hair dye formulations. They stated, however, that in view of the paucity of human studies, that while they saw no reason to make patients feel it was obligatory, they did feel that, given the seriousness of the risk—however small—it would be best for women to avoid hair dye and permanents during the first trimester of pregnancy. However, they concluded that "it is a big leap from there to a suggestion that all pregnant beauticians or beauticians contemplating pregnancy quit their jobs."

Where does one draw the line between being too cautious and too casual? Obviously, there is no easy answer to that question. The lack of general consensus leaves this matter open to the inclination of the individual physician and/or the patient. But keep one thing in mind: Just because one of the ingredients in a prescription or over-the-counter preparation

> **Check with your doctor before using prescription strength topical creams, lotions, and ointments during pregnancy.**

has the potential for toxicity doesn't mean that the product is toxic. Toxicity is a matter of degree of concentration and is related to the total amount ingested and to individual susceptibility. Take, for example, a compound called phenol. When ingested or absorbed in large quantities, phenol can cause kidney or heart failure. A form of phenol called hexylresorcinol is found in mouthwashes. There-fore, no pregnant woman should use mouthwash, right? Wrong. Hexylresorcinol is used in .001 percent concentrations in mouth-wash. It takes a 2 percent concentration (or two thousand times that dosage) to cause problems. It's the same for many other compounds as well.

Nursing Mothers and Medication Use

In general, drugs given to a nursing mother pose less risk to her baby than what they pose during pregnancy to the gestating em-bryo or fetus. The amount of drug appearing in breast milk is sel-dom more than 1 to 2 percent of the dose taken by the mother. This amount is usually not hazardous to the nursing infant. But, if you must take a potentially hazardous drug while you are breast-feeding, to reduce its impact, take the medication directly *after* breast-feeding and avoid nursing for as long a time as possible. And be sure that your baby's doctor knows and approves of your nursing the baby while you are taking that drug.

> Drugs given to a nursing mother pose less risk to her baby than to a fetus during pregnancy.

There are no skin-related drugs that are strictly contraindi-cated in nursing mothers, but tetracycline and high-dose estrogens should be avoided if at all possible. Contraceptives, antihistamines, and corticosteroids appear to be safe in breast-feeding mothers.

The skin irritation and rashes that sometimes develop around the nipple from breast-feeding presents an additional problem for treatment: how to apply a cream or ointment to the affected area without the baby ingesting the medication while nursing. The usual method is to spread the medication on the breast after breast-feeding and to wipe the breast clean before the next feeding. This will minimize the amount of medication taken in by the baby.

The Effect of Pregnancy on the Skin, Hair, and Nails

Pregnancy affects every layer of the skin and affects the hair and nails as well. Sometimes its effects are desirable—like thicker, more luxuriant hair. Sometimes they can signal problems, and sometimes they are just simply changes, normal to pregnancy but noticeably different from the way your skin, hair, or nails looked or behaved when you were not pregnant. This section will attempt to sort all this out by discussing the impact of pregnancy on the skin and the way it functions (the impact on the oil glands or skin elasticity, for example) and its effect on the hair and nails.

Skin Pigmentation in Pregnancy

The most common skin change seen during pregnancy is called hyperpigmentation. This is a darkening of the skin. Usually, the skin darkens in just a few areas—those parts of the body that already have a lot of pigment to begin with, like the nipples, the areola (the area surrounding the nipples), the genital area, and the armpits. Up to 90 percent of pregnant women, regardless of their skin color, will experience darkening in these areas of the body. It is, however, rare for pregnant women to get darker all over. When widespread hyperpigmentation does occur, it is usually related to a thyroid problem, and pre-existing thyroid disorders have been known to be aggravated by pregnancy. Any pregnant woman who develops a generalized darkening of the skin should have her thyroid gland checked.

Hyperpigmentation fades somewhat after delivery, but some degree of darkening always remains. Darker-skinned women will experience more hyperpigmentation than fair-skinned women do.

Why is skin pigment affected in this way during pregnancy? At first, scientists thought that a certain hormone, called melanocyte-stimulating hormone (MSH), was the culprit. As its name implies, this hormone stimulates the melanocytes, which are the cells of the skin that produce pigment. Since the early studies indicated that pregnant women had higher levels of MSH in their bloodstream than nonpregnant women did, it was only logical to assume that MSH was the cause of the hyperpigmentation found in pregnancy. Alas, things were not as simple as that. Apparently, the mechanism of turning up the pigment cells of the skin is more involved. To make a long story short, most investigators now feel that estrogen and possibly progesterone are the main stimulators of melanocytes. This is supported by the fact that women taking birth control pills can develop the same signs of hyperpigmentation that pregnant women do.

> **Darker-skinned women will experience more hyperpigmentation than fair-skinned women do.**

Linea Nigra

In most pregnant women, a dark line develops from the lower chest down to the pubic area. This streak is called the linea nigra, which is Latin for "dark line." It tends to go away after pregnancy.

Melasma

Be on the lookout for a condition that develops in about three out of four pregnant women. It is called melasma, but it's also known as the "mask of pregnancy." This, because it takes on the appearance of a mask—the skin on the upper cheeks develop a dark color and, sometimes, so does the forehead and upper lip. Melasma may last for months or years after pregnancy. Its cause remains a mystery. Hormones and sunlight may play a role. In fact, nonpregnant women taking birth control pills have been known to develop melasma, too.

If you have olive-colored skin, you will have more of a tendency to develop melasma. Treatment can be quite frustrating.

Laser techniques lighten melasma by up to 50 percent or more.

Bleaching creams may offer some improvement, but they take months to work and can be irritating to the skin. Retin-A, alone or together with bleaching creams, is of some help as well. Perhaps the most promising treatment of all are the newer laser techniques. These lighten melasma by up to 50 percent or more.

On rare occasions men can develop melasma. What causes a man's skin to act like a pregnant woman's skin? The reasons are unclear, but in a study that I conducted on ten such men it appeared that heredity might have played a role.

Skin Glands in Pregnancy

The Eccrine Glands

Eccrine (sweat) glands help to regulate the body's temperature. Eccrine activity increases in the final months of pregnancy, resulting in an increase in sweating in the last trimester. The reason for this is unclear. Some physicians feel that because of the marked weight gain during the last months of pregnancy the body sweats more. Others have attributed it to increased activity of the thyroid gland. Whatever the cause, this increase in sweating makes pregnant women more susceptible to developing *miliaria*, which are tiny whiteheads on the skin caused by a plugging up of the sweat glands. *Dyshidrotic eczema*, a sweat-related skin rash, is also seen with increased frequency in pregnancy.

Only one part of the body sweats less during pregnancy: the palms. Why is that so? It is felt to be related to certain complicated interactions with the adrenal glands.

Sebaceous Glands

Sebaceous glands are the oil wells of the skin and serve to lubricate it. Oil gland activity, like sweat gland activity, increases during pregnancy, although the pattern of increase is not the same for each woman. Some women experience a marked rise in sebaceous activity in the last trimester, while others experience different and more irregular patterns. But whatever the course sebaceous gland activity takes, oily skin is a common complaint during pregnancy. After delivery, things return to their normal state.

Doctors are at a loss to explain this increase in sebaceous gland activity. It has been shown that small amounts of estrogen inhibit oil production, and with all of the estrogen circulating during pregnancy, you'd think that sebaceous glands would turn off. But this is clearly not the case.

Specific oil glands exist on the skin of the breast. During the first two months of pregnancy, these sebaceous glands enlarge and form small bumps around the nipple. The glands are called Montgomery's tubercles. Their appearance is so reliable that many physicians believe that you can tell if a woman is pregnant just by examining her breasts. A woman once came into my office complaining that she was developing brown bumps around her nipples. Instead of giving her a prescription for a cream, I ordered a pregnancy test. It turned out to be positive. This was one of the few instances where a dermatologist recognized the pregnancy before the obstetrician did. Montgomery's tubercles shrink back to their pre-pregnancy size after delivery.

Skin Elasticity

The stretch marks of pregnancy, or *striae gravidarum*, are the result of the slow but steady stretching of the elastic fibers of the skin. It is estimated that almost 90 percent of pregnant women have some stretch marks. These marks usually do not become evident until the latter part of pregnancy, but, depending upon how rapidly the body grows and the skin expands, they can occur earlier. The most commonly affected areas are the breasts and the abdomen. In White women, the stretch marks initially assume a pink or purple color due to the fact that the underlying blood vessels show through the thinned out (stretched out) skin. With time, the color fades, leaving a whitish color. In African Americans, the initial color is a dark brown that gradually fades to a lighter brown. In both groups, the skin never recovers its full thickness but always remains thinned out to some extent.

> **Almost 90 percent of pregnant women develop some stretch marks.**

Treatments? I (and others) have had some success with Retin-A. Improvement rather than total cure is the rule. I have had some women tell me that vitamin E oil has helped them, although this has not been subjected to any scientific evaluation. Stretch marks are not unique to pregnancy. They also occur when the skin stretches due to rapid weight gain, or in weightlifters, where muscle build-up stretches the skin.

Blood Vessels in Pregnancy

Pregnancy has a very distinct effect on blood vessels: as the circulatory system adapts to serve both the pregnant woman and the fetus, the blood vessels tend to grow rapidly.

Varicose Veins

One of the most common and noticeable results of the rapid growth of blood vessels is the development of varicose, or dilated, veins in the legs. These may be superficial or deep.

The superficial ones are mostly cosmetic problems. Some of the deeper ones can be serious. Blood clots can form in them, with accompanying pain in the calf. Fortunately, this is a rare occurrence, but the results can be fatal.

When the veins of the thigh become blocked, a milky white streak can form. This is known as *phlegmasia alba dolens*. This is reasonably rare and corrects itself after delivery. Fortunately, the most common type are the superficial varicose veins—the kind that are visible through the surface of the skin. They can assume several patterns: squiggly red or blue lines may appear on the thighs and legs or closely grouped veins that radiate in all directions (often referred to as a "starburst" pattern). Unfortunately, most of the superficial varicose veins tend to persist even after pregnancy if they are untreated.

Sclerotherapy, also known as varicose vein injections, remains the treatment of choice for superficial venous varicosities. This is done after the pregnancy. The medication that is injected into the veins in sclerotherapy can be one of many different preparations— sodium chloride, sodium morrhuate, sodium sotradecol, or aethoxysklerol. Some are more painful, some carry higher risks of side effects. Every varicose vein specialist develops an affinity for one particular solution and sticks with it. Sclerotherapy can clear up to 80 percent of varicose veins. Possible side effects, though uncommon, include pigment spots and superficial ulcers (see chapter 6).

> **Most of the superficial varicose veins tend to persist even after pregnancy.**

Facial veins may also enlarge during pregnancy. Until a few years ago, sclerotherapy was the treatment of choice for these as well. But, on the face, this type of treatment presented several problems. There was more pain, more chance of complications, and a lower success rate than when used on leg veins. Another method—electric needle burning—had some success but often caused scarring. Then the pulsed dye laser came along. This laser emits a specialized light beam that hones in on blood vessels only. It passes through the upper layers of skin without damaging them and is selectively absorbed by red blood vessels, which are superficial dilated vessels. When treated by this method they "pop" and disintegrate, leaving the skin clear once again. Each dye laser "zap," referred to as a pulse, feels like the snap of a rubber band. It leaves the treated skin black and blue for about a week before fading out. Larger vessels may take several treatments to eradicate. (See chapter 6.)

The Spider Nevus

One of the more noticeable blood vessel problems of pregnancy is the spider nevus. In its center is a red dot that often pulsates. This represents the "feeder" artery that supplies the "legs" of the spider. These are the long, skinny blood vessels that lead away from the central dot. The entire spider nevus is surrounded by an area of redness. Spider nevi can appear anywhere on the body. Two out of every three pregnant women develop a spider nevus. The

> **Two out of every three pregnant women develop a spider nevus.**

incidence in nonpregnant women is only 10 percent. The most frequently affected areas are the neck, face, and arms. Spider nevi enlarge as the pregnancy progresses. Most go away within two months postpartum, but up to 25 percent may persist. A small-needle electric current will usually eradicate them. Pulsed dye laser treatment is another treatment that works.

Palmar Erythema

Pregnant women often notice that the palms of their hands are much redder during pregnancy; sometimes they are bright red, sometimes red with a bluish tinge. This condition, called palmar erythema, is present in 62 percent of pregnant women who are White. The incidence in pregnant African American women is much less, only 35 percent. As the pregnancy progresses, the color becomes more pronounced. Within the first two months after delivery the palms revert back to their normal color. The same condition can occur in people with cirrhosis of the liver or with hyperthyroidism. In each of these conditions, including pregnancy, an increased sensitivity to estrogens is the suspected cause. And although skin color is what is noticeable about this condition, it is not related to the pigmentation changes associated with pregnancy (discussed earlier in the chapter). Instead, it results from the effects pregnancy can produce on the blood vessels.

> Palmar Erythema is present in 62 percent of pregnant women who are White but in only 35 percent who are African American.

Raynaud's Phenomenon

The blood vessel changes that take place during pregnancy can have a beneficial effect as well. Women with Raynaud's phenomenon—a condition in which the blood vessels of the fingers are always contracted—experience marked improvement. Ordinarily, the blood vessel contraction means that blood cannot flow easily, and this gives the fingertips a bluish color. The normally poor circulation associated with Raynaud's phenomenon can cause great pain, especially if cold weather or cold water further constrict the blood vessels. This is why the dilation of blood vessels associated with pregnancy provides welcome relief for women with this condition. Unfortunately, this beneficial change is limited to the pregnancy. As with other blood vessel conditions, things go back to their pre-pregnancy state soon after delivery.

> Women with Raynaud's phenomenon experience marked improvement during pregnancy.

Cutis Marmorata

Some pregnant women are disconcerted to find a purple waffle pattern developing on their thighs. It's called cutis marmorata. This condition comes and goes and seems to be due to the constriction and dilation of the blood vessels. Cutis marmorata is totally benign.

Hemangiomas

When tiny blood vessels are packed closely together, they form bright red bumps called hemangiomas. These can vary in size from a pinhead to a marble. Despite their striking red appearance, hemangiomas never bleed. Pregnant women may develop tens to hundreds of these small bumps. In addition, hemangiomas that are present at the beginning of pregnancy may grow bigger. Most of them fade out after the baby is born. Hemangiomas may be burned off, cut off, or lasered off.

> Pregnant women may develop tens to hundreds of small bright red bumps called hemangiomas.

The Gums in Pregnancy

Although the gums are not usually thought of as part of the skin, they are made up of mucous membrane, which is similar to skin in some respects. During pregnancy, the gums may become swollen. The process can begin during the first trimester and can progress throughout the pregnancy. In addition to swelling, the gums can become red and bleed easily. The lower gums are usually more affected than the upper gums. This condition can be painful, but infection is uncommon. Improvement occurs within the first few weeks after delivery, but there may be some residual swelling. Estrogen stimulation is thought to be the main cause of these gum problems. The gum swelling, or enlargement, is also attributed to the increase in the blood volume that takes place during pregnancy.

> During pregnancy, the gums may become swollen.

There are other conditions, unrelated to pregnancy, that can cause gum problems. Scurvy (lack of vitamin C) leads to gum bleeding and fragility. Leukemia may cause similar symptoms. Finally, the anti-epileptic drug phenytoin (Dilantin) is notorious as a cause of overgrown gums. All of these other potential causes must be considered when deciding why a pregnant woman is having gum problems. Not everything that happens during pregnancy is due to pregnancy.

Pyogenic Granuloma

In about 2 percent of pregnant women, there develops something that has come to be known as the "pregnancy tumor." Its scientific name is pyogenic granuloma. It is a proliferation of gum tissue in a localized area that molds itself into a bright red bump. These can bleed easily. Although the pregnancy tumor usually regresses postpartum, the constant pain, bleeding, or irritation may be reason enough to have it removed before delivery. As in the case of other vascular growths, excision or destruction cures the tumor—it doesn't grow back.

The Hair

Most pregnant women claim that their hair seems thicker and more luxuriant. Scientific evidence supports those observations. Studies have shown that the actual number of growing hairs increases during pregnancy, and fewer are shed. The hairs themselves are not any thicker, there are just more of them, which is why the coiffure looks and is fuller.

Pregnant women have thicker and more luxurious hair because the actual number of growing hairs increases during pregnancy, and fewer are shed.

The growing hairs are called anagen hairs (see chapter 2). The anagen phase continues until the end of pregnancy. When the anagen phase ends, the telogen phase begins. Telogen hairs are in a resting pattern. So a good number of the anagen, or growing, hairs fall out after pregnancy. This hair loss usually does not become apparent until two to three months after delivery.

The thinning out of the scalp hair is called *telogen effluvium*. Telogen effluvium usually lasts for a few months. Then the hairs go back to their regular growing and resting cycle and everything gets back to normal. However, some women don't experience regrowth for up to a year. A very small percentage will be permanently left with thinned out hair. When this occurs, the frontal hairline and the crown of the scalp are the most commonly affected areas. (See chapter 2.)

Childbirth, like anything that stresses the body, emotionally or physically, can cause hair to fall out after delivery.

Anything that stresses the body, emotionally or physically, can cause hair to fall out. Severe illness, auto accidents, and operations are some physical causes. Divorce or losing a job are events that can cause emotional stress. You can just imagine where pregnancy fits into all of this. Pregnancy, the tremendous physical effort of childbirth, and all the worries of raising that baby, each by itself or taken together, are enough to make anyone's hair fall out!

Until recently there was nothing to do for hair loss except to hope for the best. The introduction of topical minoxidil (Rogaine) several years ago provided a breakthrough. Tests with newer hair-growing drugs are being conducted. Pregnancy-related hair loss mostly occurs *after* pregnancy. But, if you do experience any hair loss while still pregnant, you must check to see if your physician feels that treating this problem is safe before you actually deliver. Rogaine is a category C drug for use during pregnancy, and all drugs, including topical ones, must be carefully considered before using them during pregnancy. (See chapters 2 and 7.)

Hirsutism (Excess Body Hair)

Excess body hair, also called hirsutism, occurs in many women, whether or not they are pregnant, but pregnancy is one of the physiological states that stimulates body hair growth. For most pregnant women, the degree of hirsutism is very mild. However, the women who are most prone to the thickest growth during pregnancy are those who, before pregnancy, tended to have more body hair than other women.

The areas of the body that are most commonly affected are the upper lip, the cheeks, and the chin. Sometimes the arms, legs, and the back experience increased hair growth also. Hirsutism goes away after delivery for most women. However, for some, the hirsutism that comes with pregnancy remains and does not reverse itself.

When hirsutism is accompanied by a bad case of acne, be aware. The combination of excess hair, bad acne, and a deepening voice signal trouble. The most common cause of these signs and symptoms in pregnancy is a disease of the ovaries. It is called *polycystic ovary disease (POD)*. POD can affect the fetus as well as the mother. In extreme cases, still-

> The combination of excess hair on the face, bad acne, and a deepening voice signal polycystic ovary disease.

births, malformations, and masculinizing changes in baby girls have been reported. POD can occur in nonpregnant women as well; in fact, it is a major cause of infertility.

The Nails

Female hormones accelerate nail growth. That's why nails grow faster in the premenstrual phase of the nonpregnant woman's cycle. With all of the extra hormones floating around during pregnancy, you'd expect the nails to grow faster during the entire nine months. But the pattern is irregular. During the first few months of pregnancy, the nails grow somewhat more rapidly than usual. The rate of growth levels off in the middle trimester. Then, during the last month of pregnancy, the nails grow much faster than ever before—about twice as fast as they normally do. After delivery, when the hormone levels drop back to normal, the nails assume their regular growth pattern again. If there is insufficient caloric intake during pregnancy nail growth can become stunted or inhibited. As discussed in chapter 2, the nails can often reflect a good bit about what is going on in the body and should be used as an indicator of problems in pregnancy as well.

> **During the last month of pregnancy, the nails grow much faster.**

Nail Problems in Pregnancy

Besides the change in rate of their growth, nails may exhibit any number of irregularities during pregnancy. Lines or furrows may run across the width of the nail. This is called *transverse grooving*. It happens when the matrix at the bottom of the nail alternately speeds up and then slows down the production of keratin. Similarly, white lines may appear as a result of the same process. Depending on what is happening in the matrix, nails may become brittle or soft. Splitting at the tips of the nails is a condition known as *distal onycholysis*. There may also be a build-up of debris or dead skin underneath the nails. This is referred to as *subungual hyperkeratosis*.

These nail problems and others will slowly clear up after delivery, although it may take as long as a year. For those disorders that do not improve, medical intervention may be necessary.

Nail problems are perhaps the most difficult area of dermatology to treat. Nails grow slowly and, as a result, respond slowly, if at all, to therapy. Certain topical creams and solutions can strengthen the split tips of distal onycholysis. Urea is a favorite ingredient in these remedies. Subungual hyperkeratosis can be dealt with in a number of ways. Trimming back the overlying nail and scraping

> **The CO_2 laser can offer a cure for a variety of nail disorders.**

out the underlying debris is helpful. Solutions such as thymol help to cement the new nail to the nail bed. The CO_2 laser can offer a cure for a variety of nail disorders. Ingrown nails, split nails, and thick nails can all be treated by an expert CO_2 laser surgeon. These methods are all safe to use during pregnancy.

Pregnancy and Pre-Existing Skin Diseases and Conditions

A woman who already has a skin condition when she becomes pregnant, quite understandably, wonders whether it will affect her pregnancy *or* her baby. She also wonders if the pregnancy will affect the skin condition.

Unfortunately, with many skin conditions it is not always clear what will happen, because so many things can be at work. Certain aspects of the disease or condition itself might interact with the woman's particular physiological characteristics, her general state of health, and the idiosyncrasies of each pregnancy. These changes and their interactions are not easily predictable but can affect the skin. And, then, there are the considerable hormonal changes associated with pregnancy that can also affect many skin conditions. In addition to hormonal change, important immunological changes are necessary to maintaining a pregnancy. For, normally, the job of the immune system is to reject what is foreign to the body. That's how it fights off infection and toxins. But, in pregnancy, the immune system has to adjust in order to accept the developing fetus, which it might otherwise regard as foreign (and thus attempt to reject). And, these immunological changes can also have considerable impact on the skin.

All these factors—which can operate together in complex and variable ways—make it difficult to predict what will happen with a pre-existing condition in any particular pregnancy. For example, the very same skin condition can be adversely affected by pregnancy in one woman and actually improve in another woman. What is yet more confounding is that the very skin condition that improves during one pregnancy in a particular woman can get worse for that same woman during the course of another of her pregnancies!

But not all is chaos. There *are* some patterns and there *is* a body of clinical evidence that allow certain generalizations to be made and certain guidelines to be suggested.

Some of the diseases mentioned below are reasonably common ones—like acne or psoriasis. Some are not very common at all but when added together affect enough women that they deserve the attention given the more common ones. Whether the condition or disease is common or rare, for each, I will discuss how pregnancy affects its course, whether pregnancy places any limits on its treatment, and how the condition affects the pregnant women or the gestating embryo or fetus.

The general and basic details about each of the diseases—all of which can occur in the nonpregnant population—appear elsewhere in the book, especially in the final chapter. *Thus, to get a more complete description of each of these diseases and conditions, please turn to chapter 8, and also check the index.*

And do be aware that since every pregnant woman, and every pregnancy that each woman experiences, is different, one cannot offer blanket statements as to the "right" way to treat each of the following skin diseases that might occur in pregnancy. The safest thing to do is check with your doctor regarding treatment of any skin condition during pregnancy.

Acne in Pregnancy

Pregnancy often occurs during early adulthood, when acne tends to be so prevalent, but the effect of pregnancy on acne is unpredictable. Sometimes it improves, sometimes it gets worse. The unpredictability is so striking that some women's acne will get worse in one pregnancy and improve in another. Or vice versa. What causes this variation is still a mystery. It might very

Acne that gets worse during pregnancy will get better after delivery.

well be due to differences in hormonal levels, or in the patterns of hormonal variation that take place between different women, or between pregnancies in the same woman. The clinical experience with birth control medication and its relationship to acne supports this explanation for the variation in acne between pregnancies. Birth control pills differ in the amount of estrogen they contain, and some types aggravate acne while others improve it.

The one clear-cut statement that can be made about acne and pregnancy is a happy one. For those whose acne gets worse during pregnancy, there is a marked improvement after delivery.

The major dilemma that acne in pregnancy poses is over whether or not to treat it. Since nobody ever died of acne, and pregnancy is a time to be cautious with medications, many physicians and patients opt for a very conservative approach. On the other hand, since permanent scarring can occur from bad acne, some physicians advocate a more aggressive approach. A decision then has to be made concerning what that treatment approach should be.

Some antibiotics used to treat acne, such as tetracycline and minocycline, are contraindicated during pregnancy because they discolor the baby's teeth and bones. But others, such as penicillin derivatives or erythromycin, are usually regarded as safe. Other treatments, like topical benzoyl peroxide and topical antibiotics, are considered by most experts to be safe to use in pregnancy. Retin-A is a bit more controversial, but there have never been any reports of problems with its use by pregnant women. In fact, a 1993 study in the respected British medical journal *Lancet* showed that using Retin-A during the first trimester of pregnancy was *not* associated with any increased incidence of congenital abnormalities.

The powerful drug Accutane is absolutely contraindicated and should never be considered in pregnancy. It is known to cause death or malformations in the fetus.

P*soriasis*

Pregnancy has no effect on the majority of women who have psoriasis. However, about one-third of pregnant women actually improve, while a small number of women experience a worsening. In addition, pregnant women who have a related condition, psoriatic arthritis, can show improvement as well. Many therapies exist for psoriasis, but many of them are not advisable to use in pregnancy. Therapy depends upon the severity of the condition. Topical steroids can be used on small areas. Ultraviolet therapy appears to be safe also. However, some of the more powerful oral medications such as methotrexate or etretinate are, for the most part, contraindicated.

M*oles,* F*reckles,* L*entigines* (Liver Spots)

Moles, or nevi, as they are known in medical parlance, tend to get larger during pregnancy. New moles can appear also. Some moles darken in color, prompting many women to seek medical at-

tention to determine if they are cancerous or on their way to becoming so. Taking that precaution is wise. For, even though during pregnancy most moles do not undergo malignant change, an occasional one does (see discussion of malignant melanoma below).

The moles that have either grown larger or darkened during pregnancy return to their pre-pregnancy state after delivery, but sometimes they retain the changes they took on during pregnancy. Freckles and lentigines, the so-called liver spots (which are not related to the liver at all), behave similarly.

Just why moles, freckles, and liver spots grow during pregnancy is not fully understood, but it is felt that estrogen is very much a factor. It has been demonstrated that moles have receptor sites on their cells for estrogen. The cells of the mole are probably stimulated when the receptor sites are bombarded by estrogen during pregnancy. When the stimulus dies down after pregnancy, the cells tend to revert back to their normal state.

If, during pregnancy, a mole is at all suggestive of becoming cancerous, or already looks cancerous, the ex-

amining physician will recommend removing it, just as at all other times in life. The procedure is quick, safe in pregnancy, and may be a lifesaver.

Skin Tags

Skin tags are just what the name implies—little tags of skin that protrude above the skin's surface. They are very common in pregnancy. Not only can new ones appear, but pre-existing ones can enlarge. They most commonly occur on the sides of the neck, the armpits, and the groin. The face and chest may also be affected but not as often. The areas where they tend to grow are generally areas where skin rubs up against skin, which is often the result of the weight gain and shape changes associated with pregnancy. It's the friction created by the rubbing of the skin that stimulates skin tag growth, although other factors, such as hormones and hereditary tendencies, may be involved. The fact that skin tags are very common in obese individuals in the very same areas of the body where they occur in pregnancy lends support to the friction hypothesis.

Skin tags can be annoying as well as unsightly. They can interfere with necklaces and pendants and often are irritated by clothing. Fortunately, they never become cancerous. In fact, many shrink away after delivery although a good many of them tend to persist. Skin tags can be frozen, burned, lasered, or snipped off. The medical name for skin tags in pregnancy is *molluscum fibrosum gravidarum*.

W*arts*

Warts that are present at the beginning of pregnancy tend to grow larger. There is some question as to whether or not pregnant women are more susceptible to the development of new warts. Certain aspects of the immune response in pregnant woman are somewhat depressed, and this could account for the increased growth of warts. Warts may, however, act differently during different pregnancies. They will lie dormant during some pregnancies, and in other pregnancies in that same woman they will grow rapidly. Warts that grow on the sole of the foot—called plantar warts—can become painful and make walking difficult. The genital warts called condyloma acuminata (see chapter 8) may become sufficiently large to make vaginal delivery impossible and cesarean section necessary.

Many warts shrink after delivery, while others stay the same size. There are the various treatments available for warts. Many are safe and effective during pregnancy. Those treatments that fail to permanently get rid of warts during pregnancy work well after delivery, due to the return of the normal immune system response that takes place after pregnancy.

C*old Sores (Fever Blisters) and Genital Herpes*

The herpes virus infections on the lips (cold sores, or fever blisters) and genital herpes eruptions usually remain localized to one area (see chapter 8), but pregnancy can increase the possibility of their being disseminated to other parts of the body. Also, the genital herpes eruptions, which can also occur in the anal area, can be transmitted to the fetus, just as with other venereal diseases. This transmission takes place either through the placenta or by direct contact when the fetus passes through the birth canal. Newborns who are infected may have severe malformations of any number of organs. Thus, if a pregnant woman has either blisters or microscopic evidence of herpes simplex in the birth canal—evidence that's determined by a positive culture—cesarean section is indicated. If, however, the genital herpes simplex infection is in the latent state (you've had it before, but at the time of delivery there are no active blisters and no microscopic evidence of the virus), the fetus will not come in contact with the virus in the birth canal.

Acyclovir is the primary antiherpes drug, but it is a category C drug for use during pregnancy.

S*yphilis*

Unfortunately, there are still many cases of syphilis among pregnant women. Pregnancy does not seem to alter the overall course of the disease, but it may aggravate some of the internal manifestations of the disease that were already present at the time of pregnancy.

The most devastating effects of syphilis in pregnancy are on the fetus. The central factor in determining whether or not the fetus will be affected has to do with when the pregnant woman became infected. Infection during the first trimester carries the worst prognosis for the fetus, while infection acquired during the last trimester may not affect the fetus or newborn at all. However, of those fetuses that are infected, one-quarter will die in their mother's womb as a result of the disease. Another quarter die shortly after birth. Those who are infected and survive need immediate antibiotic treatment to halt the disease.

> **Syphilis carries the worst prognosis for the fetus during the first three months of pregnancy.**

Interestingly, in pregnant women who had untreated syphilis for five years or more before the pregnancy, there is less likelihood of transmitting the disease to the fetus than in women who acquired syphilis during pregnancy. Apparently this has to do with the stage the infection is in when the fetus is subjected to it.

As with syphilis in the rest of the population, injections of penicillin remain the mainstay of syphilis therapy in pregnant women. One problem emerging in the treatment of syphilis in pregnancy results from the fact that the organism that causes syphilis is beginning to show some resistance to the penicillin. However, the alternative treatment, oral tetracycline, which is curative in high doses, is not a viable treatment during pregnancy because it can discolor the baby's teeth and bones.

Syphilis can be diagnosed either by direct observation or by blood tests, depending on the stage it's in. Despite this, the number of cases of syphilis increases each year. Prompt diagnosis and treatment are the most important factors in determining a good outcome. However, too many cases are slipping by, undiagnosed.

Keloids

Keloids are overgrown scars. In line with the fact that everything grows in pregnancy, keloids are no exception. Somehow, pregnancy stimulates existing keloids to enlarge. Although some keloids may shrink back to their pre-pregnancy size after delivery, most of them remain enlarged. If someone with a history of keloids has a cesarean section, keloids often form at the incision site.

Firm compresses and/or injections of cortisone into the keloids are the treatments of choice.

Malignant Melanoma

Pregnancy has a definite effect upon the prognosis, or outcome, of malignant melanoma. The melanomas tend to grow more rapidly. This increases the ability of the cancer to metastasize, or spread. The deeper the melanomas, the more rapidly they grow.

That pregnancy worsens melanoma is of considerable significance because one-third of all the people who develop a melanoma are women of childbearing age. The factor linking pregnancy to melanoma is probably estrogen. Malignant melanomas have a large number of receptors on their cells for estrogen, and the increased

Pregnancy worsens melanoma and can be spread to the fetus.

levels of estrogen in the blood during pregnancy tend to stimulate the melanoma cells to grow. To add to the problem, malignant melanoma is one of the very few cancers that can actually spread from the mother to the fetus during the course of pregnancy. Therefore, it is possible for a baby to be born with melanoma.

Thus, being vigilant about new or changing moles is one of the most important things that a woman and her physician can do during the course of a pregnancy. Aggressive surgical and some-times chemotherapeutical measures may be necessary in advanced cases. In smaller melanomas, simple excisions usually suffice.

A*canthosis Nigricans*

Acanthosis nigricans, a condition that occurs both in Whites and in Blacks, is a darkening of the skin, usually around the neck and at the armpits. It can occur in conjunction with a number of diseases and conditions—including cancer, diabetes insipidus, pregnancy, and obesity. In the nonpregnant individual acanthosis nigricans may make its appearance before, or at the time of, or after the onset of the disease it accompanies. However, when it develops in pregnancy (and obesity), acanthosis nigricans always occurs *after* the onset of these conditions.

As one might expect, the skin darkening slowly disappears after pregnancy, although there tend to be recurrences in subse-quent pregnancies. There is no relationship between the outcome of the pregnancy and acanthosis nigricans.

L*upus*

Pregnancy does not seem to have any major effect upon the discoid form of lupus—the kind of lupus that involves only the skin—but the same cannot be said for the systemic variety. In systemic lupus, pregnancy tends to worsen the skin rash that accompanies lupus, and the internal organs suffer as well. When the kidneys are diseased by lupus, the fetus is at particularly high risk, especially after de-livery. Hazards to the fetus include low birth weight and a higher than average risk of death. On occasion, a newborn will itself have some of the manifestations of lupus, such as a skin rash or heart disease.

In systemic lupus, pregnancy tends to worsen the lupus skin rash.

Given the relatively high incidence of lupus in women of childbearing age and the potential for severe complications to both mother and child, early recognition of symptoms and the close monitoring of this condition by a physician are essential.

D*ermatomyositis*

Dermatomyositis involves both the skin and the muscles. The most characteristic skin feature is the so-called heliotrope rash. The muscles become increasingly weak and sore, especially the shoulder and hip muscles.

Most cases of dermatomyositis are not affected by pregnancy one way or the other. But it does have a considerable impact on the fetus, causing a fetal mortality rate of an astounding 46 percent.

Scleroderma

Scleroderma means "tight skin." Tightness usually begins on the fingers and hands, where the skin becomes thick and stiff. When the face is affected, there can be a loss of mobility of the skin around the mouth.

Although there appears to be somewhat of a decrease in fertility among women with scleroderma, the disease does not adversely affect pregnancy and the skin does not worsen in pregnancy. However, women with kidney disease as a result of scleroderma should be carefully watched during the course of their pregnancy.

Scleroderma is the most difficult of the collagen vascular diseases to treat. Since the basic process is sclerosis—an overthickening of the collagen and not an inflammatory process—this disease presents a therapeutic challenge to physicians. There are simply fewer treatments for this kind of problem than there are for inflammation. New types of drugs are in the development stage for scleroderma, but, as yet, there is no satisfactory current treatment.

Hansen's Disease (Leprosy)

Hansen's disease is endemic to Africa and Asia, but cases are found all over the world. Its skin signs include decreased sensation to touch and temperature, pigment changes, nodules, nerve damage, and mental changes. But which of these occurs depends on whether the disease takes the tuberculoid form or the lepromatous form.

Hansen's disease is affected adversely during the first trimester of pregnancy. After that, the effects are not as striking. The reasons for this are not well understood but are probably immunological in nature.

The drug that is most frequently used for treating this disease—Dapsone—is a category C medication, meaning that it must be used with considerable caution in pregnancy. Rifampin, an antituberculosis medicine, is a category C drug. It should be noted that the other drug used for this disease is thalidomide, but it is associated with severe birth defects and has not been available in the United States since the 1950s.

Neurofibromatosis (von Recklinghausen's Disease)

Neurofibromas are overgrowths of nerve cells in the skin, manifested by soft subcutaneous nodules. Pregnancy can trigger their growth, so it is no surprise that pregnant women with von Recklinghausen's disease experience a worsening of this condition. Because large neurofibromas can compress nerves and blood vessels, the condition can cause hypertension, which is especially risky in pregnancy. There is also an increase in stillbirths and spontaneous abortions associated with this disease. As in nonpregnant individuals, treatment consists of surgical decompression of the affected nerve or surgical removal of the offending neurofibroma.

Sarcoidosis

Sarcoidosis, or sarcoid, is a disorder that can affect many organs in the body, notably the skin, lungs, and the lymph glands. The basic defect is a depression of immune function of the T-cells of the body. Since this disease responds to immunosuppressive drugs, such as high dose steroids and azathioprine, perhaps the natural immunosuppression of pregnancy—which occurs so that the mother's body won't treat the fetus as a foreign object and reject it—provides a kind of temporary "treatment." The use of conventional medical treatments should be discussed at length with your doctor, since the powerful drugs that may be used to treat sarcoidosis can carry significant risk to the mother or fetus.

> **Pregnancy provides a kind of temporary "treatment" for sarcoidosis.**

Ehlers-Danlos Syndrome

Ehlers-Danlos syndrome involves an inherited defect in collagen formation, affecting the skin, bones, and the blood vessels. It is characterized by hyperextensibility of the skin—the skin can be pulled high up and away from the underlying muscles—which means that the skin can become baggy in some areas or bruise easily in others. Wound healing is impaired, wrinkles are common, bones are easily dislocated, joints may become loose, the blood vessels can become very fragile, and the arteries may tear easily.

The course of pregnancy in women with Ehlers-Danlos syndrome is variable. The skin problems associated with this condition tend to be unaffected, and most women do well throughout their pregnancy. However, some women may develop extensive vaginal skin lacerations because the skin tears easily during delivery. This can result in hemorrhage, and wounds heal quite slowly in women with this syndrome. In view of this potentially serious complication, it behooves every pregnant women with any type of Ehlers-Danlos syndrome to be followed carefully by her physician throughout the pregnancy. Since, at present, there is no effective therapy for Ehlers-Danlos syndrome, treatment consists of taking good care of its symptoms, like preventing and carefully treating skin infections.

> **Women with Ehlers-Danlos syndrome may develop extensive vaginal skin lacerations during delivery.**

Hidradenitis Suppurativa

Hidradenitis suppurativa is a chronic skin disease affecting the apocrine glands of the armpits and groin areas. The glands in these areas become inflamed and drain pus.

The course of hidradenitis suppurativa during pregnancy varies, but most women tend to improve. It has been shown that apocrine gland secretions decrease during the last months of pregnancy, and this fact may account for the improvement seen then. The improvement, however, is short-lived, and relapses are the rule after delivery. And not every woman does better during pregnancy. Some cases involving the groin area can deteriorate to such a degree that regular vaginal delivery is impossible, and a cesarean section is indicated.

Pemphigus

Pemphigus is an uncommon but potentially fatal skin disease. It consists of numerous large blisters that can form anywhere on the skin or mucous membranes, such as the mouth or genitalia. The medical literature indicates that pemphigus doesn't have an undermining effect on pregnancy or labor, although pregnancy makes pemphigus worse. While the specific reason for this is not known, we do know that it is an autoimmune disease, and autoimmune diseases are affected by pregnancy.

Pregnancy-related flares in this condition involve an increase in blistering, usually noticed in the first or second trimesters. Some women even experience a worsening after delivery. While certain women are affected in each and every pregnancy, others are affected only in some of their pregnancies. Obviously, pregnant women with pemphigus should receive very close, careful medical care because of the potentially serious consequences of the disease.

As with lupus, oral steroids are required for control of pemphigus. Fortunately, because it is usually a disease of the sixth and seventh decades of life, its appearance in pregnant women is rare.

Acrodermatitis Enteropathica

This uncommon familial disorder is characterized by severe blistering and a pustular rash around the orifices of the body (the mouth, anus, and vagina), an eczematous type of red, scaly rash on the hands and feet and, occasionally, bald patches on the scalp. Marked diarrhea and malabsorption can be present also.

Acrodermatitis enteropathica tends to get worse with pregnancy, with flare-ups usually occurring in the early rather than in the latter part of pregnancy. But the condition dramatically clears up within a week after delivery.

The usual treatment for this condition—zinc supplements—are generally considered safe for use in pregnancy.

Hermansky-Pudlak Syndrome

Hermansky-Pudlak syndrome involves a loss of pigment in the skin, decreased color in the iris of the eye, and a defect in the clotting cells of the blood—the platelets. As one can imagine, a clotting disorder can make pregnancy risky, but several reported pregnancies in patients with Hermansky-Pudlak syndrome have transpired without major complications. The skin and eye components of the syndrome were unaffected by the pregnancy.

Pseudoxanthoma Elasticum

Pseudoxanthoma elasticum involves a degeneration of elastic tissue. As a result, all organs of the body that contain elastic tissue can be affected: the skin, retina, blood vessels, gastrointestinal tract, and the heart. There is no indication that women with pseudoxanthoma elasticum have any impairment of fertility. And the yellowish pebble-like bumps, which are its characteristic skin signs, do not increase in number or in size during pregnancy. However, because of the effect of this condition on the blood vessels, and because the blood vessels have to work harder during pregnancy, pseudoxanthoma elasticum poses significant risks to the pregnant woman—risks like gastrointestinal bleeding and congestive heart failure. With this in mind, it is important to diagnose this disease before pregnancy. The most common way to establish the diagnosis is by examining the skin symptoms. Whenever a woman with this disease becomes pregnant, she should be under close medical care throughout the course of her pregnancy.

> Pseudoxanthoma elasticum poses significant risks to the pregnant woman, so it is important to diagnose this disease before pregnancy.

Porphyria Cutanea Tarda

Porphyria cutanea tarda involves a number of skin signs, including excessive facial hair extending from the eyebrows to the temples, blisters on the sun-exposed areas of the hands and arms, and scarring where the deeper blisters heal. Because birth control pills with a high estrogen content seem to cause flare-ups in this condition, it would stand to reason that pregnancy, with its wide swings in hormonal levels, might have a similar effect. However, this does not appear to be the case. Pregnant women with porphyria cutanea tarda do fairly well, with only a mild worsening of their skin condition. However, pregnant women with the *internal* types of porphyria, namely acute intermittent porphyria and variegate porphyria, have a much more difficult course and must be watched very closely by their physicians. Severe cases of these forms of porphyria, when exacerbated by pregnancy, can result in death.

Henoch-Schonlein Purpura

The classic presentation of this disease is the sudden onset of purplish red patches and bumps on the legs, buttocks, and sometimes the arms. These are caused by bleeding in the skin. Bleeding in internal organs, such as the gastrointestinal tract and kidneys, can occur as well. Women who develop Henoch-Schonlein purpura for the first time during the course of their pregnancy appear to do all right as long as they are under good medical care.

Histiocytosis X

Histiocytosis X is a generic term for three rare diseases in which the basic defect is a proliferation of cells called histiocytes. While this condition can affect any organ, those that are most usually affected are the lungs, lymph glands, bones, hormone glands, and the skin. Only a few cases have been reported in pregnant women, and in those cases there were no flare-ups in the skin symptoms—pregnancy did *not* result in the appearance of new skin bumps, nodules, or ulcerations, or in the severity of existing ones. Pregnant women with this ailment do seem to experience problems with excessive thirst and urination—a condition called diabetes insipidus. (This is different from diabetes mellitus, which is often simply referred to as "diabetes" and is associated with elevated blood sugar.) However, patients reported doing better once the baby was born.

Tuberous Sclerosis

The multitude of skin problems associated with tuberous sclerosis tend to be unaffected by pregnancy, but the kidneys may enlarge, causing a problem with hypertension.

Skin Diseases Seen Only in Pregnancy

The innumerable changes that occur during pregnancy can result in the development of certain skin diseases that occur *only* in pregnancy. Although little is currently known about their cause, we know from clinical experience that they run the gamut from simply bothersome to potentially life-threatening to the mother and/or the fetus.

PUPPP

PUPPP is a skin disorder of pregnancy that was first recognized as a separate disease in 1979. Its odd name, PUPPP, is actually an

acronym for "pruritic urticarial papules and plaques of pregnancy." Before being viewed as a separate disease, its symptoms
were felt to represent a variant of hives or evidence of an allergy or
other conditions. It is characterized by itchy skin eruptions, which
can vary from small, red bumps to large wheals. When severe, the
rashes will often join together to form big
patches. They tend to start at the navel and
then fan out to cover the rest of the abdomen,
often appearing over the stretch marks of pregnancy that are already on the abdomen. Sometimes the rash will extend to the
thighs, arms, and buttocks. Fortunately, the face is never affected.
The itching associated with PUPPP may range from mild to mad-
dening. However the whole problem goes away after delivery.

> **PUPPP tends to appear in first pregnancies in the third trimester.**

   The cause of PUPPP is unknown. Many studies of the blood
and skin have been performed, but there are no clues as to why this
skin disease occurs. PUPPP tends to appear in the third trimester. It
also is more common in first pregnancies as opposed to subsequent
ones.

   Despite intensive investigation, there have been no reports of
fetal abnormalities associated with PUPPP. However, compared to
other pregnant women, women with PUPPP experience a significantly increased weight gain. Also, about 10 percent of the PUPPP
pregnancies have been shown to result in twin births, a percentage
that is about six times higher than the national average. Based
upon this, it has been suspected that a marked increase in weight
gain and abdominal girth play a role in the development of PUPPP.
Because PUPPP's status as a separate disease is so recent, we can
only hypothesize. A good deal of detective work still remains in order to determine all of the causative factors and consequences of
this skin malady.

   PUPPP is usually treated with oral antihistamines, which offer
symptomatic relief. Cool topical solutions may be of benefit as well.

Impetigo Herpetiformis

Although the name implies otherwise, impetigo herpetiformis is
neither a variant of impetigo nor of herpes. Instead, it is thought to
be similar to pustular psoriasis (see chapter 8), although its cause is
unknown. It is characterized by numerous pus-filled blisters that
appear in the groin and lower abdominal areas. The skin around
the breasts is affected as well. The pus in the blisters is sterile—it

contains no contagious bacteria. In severe cases, the pustules can cover the entire skin surface of the body as well as portions of the mouth. To make matters worse, fever, vomiting, and malaise can be accompanying symptoms. As you probably can surmise from this description, impetigo herpetiformis can be very serious—so much so it is sometimes fatal. In addition to the risk to the pregnant woman, there is a high fetal mortality rate. Fortunately, however, this condition is rare.

Pregnancies in which impetigo herpetiformis develop must be very closely monitored. Hospitalization along with intravenous (IV) fluids and antibiotics may be required. At term, cesarean section must be considered if the mother's debility contributes to excessive fetal distress.

Papular Dermatitis of Spangler

Spangler's dermatitis was first described in the medical literature in the early 1960s. It consists of very itchy small bumps that can appear anywhere on the skin. A characteristic feature of this skin disease is that only seven or eight new scattered bumps appear every day. Another important characteristic of this condition is that there is a low level of the hormone cortisol, which is a steroid-like hormone. But the actual connection between cortisol and Spangler's dermatitis is unclear.

The disease tends to occur at any point in the course of a pregnancy—there is no preference for any one of the trimesters. It may last several days to several months. Recurrences are common in subsequent pregnancies.

Although there does not appear to be any significant risk to the mother, the same cannot be said for the fetus. A fetal mortality rate of up to 30 percent has been reported. Early diagnosis and treatment with cortisone derivatives can be helpful, but even with appropriate therapy, the fetal risk remains high. It is important to distinguish this disorder from other similar disorders, such as scabies (which it resembles), since prompt and proper treatment may save the gestating fetus.

Prurigo Gestationis of Besnier

Prurigo gestationis of Besnier differs from Spangler's dermatitis (see immediately above) in that the bumps of Besnier appear all at once while Spangler's bumps make their appearance in a regular progression of seven to eight per day. It is important to differentiate between these two similar disorders because this one—prurigo gestationis of Besnier—is not associated with any increased risk to mother or fetus, while there is a significant fetal mortality rate with Spangler's dermatitis. Two other factors that differentiate the two diseases are that Besnier's bumps tend to occur in the second trimester and the blood level of cortisol is normal in Besnier's.

As with the other rashes of pregnancy, prurigo gestationis of Besnier goes away after delivery. However, oftentimes, a persistent dark spot will occur at the sites where the bumps had been, and these spots will remain for many months until finally fading out. As with PUPPP (see above), treatment is symptomatic. But since the itching can be quite intense, extensive use of topical steroids, or even oral steroids, may be necessary.

Autoimmune Progesterone Dermatitis

As the name suggests, this is a rash that is produced by the body's own immune reaction to progesterone, a hormone that is produced in large amounts during pregnancy. This rare condition produces acne-like lesions on the buttocks and extremities. Often there is swelling of the joints and the soft tissues. Also, a high rate of spontaneous abortions has been reported to be related to this condition.

Autoimmune progesterone dermatitis was discovered in 1973 by a dermatologist who noticed that one family seemed to be having an usually high incidence of rashes during pregnancy. After conducting some laboratory research on these patients he was able to come up with the relationship between extremely high levels of progesterone and this condition.

Pruritus Gravidarum

Generalized itching has been reported to occur in almost 20 percent of all pregnancies. Some of this itching, when severe, is considered to be evidence of the condition called pruritus gravidarum, which usually occurs during the last trimester. Surprisingly, there are no visible skin rashes or other skin symptoms. Pruritus gravidarum is felt to be related to recurrent cholestasis of pregnancy. The bile ducts tend to back up during some pregnancies, and an accumulation of bile products can cause itching all over the body.

The diagnosis is established by abnormal results on blood tests of liver function. Jaundice, a yellowing of the skin that frequently accompanies liver disorders, may or may not be present. Usually there is a strong family history of similar bouts of itching during pregnancy.

Although the itching may be intense, there is virtually no risk to the pregnant woman herself. However, this disease does carry a 13 percent rate of stillbirth or prematurity. As such, it is important to establish the diagnosis of pruritus gravidarum in order to differentiate it from other liver-related conditions that may occur during pregnancy, such as hepatitis or drug reactions. Other causes of generalized itching may include a drug or food allergy, insect bites, or hives.

Herpes Gestationis

Herpes gestationis is not caused by the herpes virus but assumes a blistering appearance similar to herpes blisters. Its incidence has been estimated as being one out of every five thousand pregnancies. It most commonly occurs in the second trimester and tends to recur in subsequent pregnancies. Although herpes gestationis is not contagious and not caused by the herpes virus, several similarities to herpes simplex exist. First, burning and itching may precede the blisters by several days. When the blisters do form, they are grouped, tense eruptions on a red base of skin. Often red rings will form, with a group of blisters on their borders. In severe cases, blisters may be large and their spread may be extensive. They may come and go in waves. Sometimes fever, nausea, and/or headache may be present. This is one of the few skin diseases of pregnancy that can be diagnosed by a skin biopsy—a characteristic microscopic pattern fluoresces when the specimen is subjected to a special light.

Needless to say, when this condition is extensive there can be significant risk of illness and sometimes even death. There appears to be some controversy as to whether or not the fetus suffers an increased risk as well. Recent reports seem to indicate that herpes gestationis is associated with an increase in prematurity and in infants who are small for their gestational age. Herpes gestationis goes away after delivery, but birth control pills or even a new menstrual cycle can precipitate recurrences. High doses of steroids will often control a severe outbreak.

One final note:

One kind of rash to be alert for if you are pregnant is one that occurs on the skin of *other* people, especially children. It is the rash of *rubella* (often called "German measles"). Many women have suffered miscarriages or borne babies with severe birth defects after being infected with rubella during pregnancy. But while the rash is a sign that the infection is present, unfortunately, children can also spread the virus *before* the rash actually appears. So, if you are pregnant but do not have immunity to German measles (either by having had the disease or the vaccination), don't just rely on the rash as a sign that rubella might be around. Keep an ear out for news of rubella cases in your community so that you can take steps to avoid exposure. If you are not pregnant but of childbearing age *and* you never had the disease as a child *or* were not immunized against it, it's wise to get the rubella vaccination. But do remember that the vaccine uses a live virus, so you should wait three to six months after being inoculated *before* becoming pregnant.

Chapter 5

Cleanliness, Care, and Cosmetics

K eeping your skin clean, healthy, and good looking is an important part of your daily routine. But, given the enormous range of soaps, cleansers, antiperspirants, sunscreens, and cosmetics to choose from, how can you decide what will work best for you? This chapter is intended to help you sort through the wide range of products, practices, and beliefs about grooming so that you will be able to decide what is best for you.

Cleanliness

How clean should your skin be? That question allows for neither a simple nor a single answer. The reason is that we have different cleaning requirements—depending on the area of the country we live in, our home and work environments, our skin's physical characteristics, and even variations in our personal standards and social expectations.

But not to worry! There are a wide variety of products to keep your skin clean. Basically, there are three types—soaps, cleanser, and detergents. (Here I will use these words in a somewhat more technical way than we do in everyday speech. So, when I speak of detergents, for example, I don't mean powders and liquids used to clean dishes and clothes; and cleansers are not the gritty powders used to scrub sinks.) All three have ingredients called surfactants. The difference between soaps, cleansers, and detergents has to do with the particular source and kind of these surfactants—and what they contribute to the cleaning process.

In soaps and detergents, the surfactants just act to abrade the skin mildly and thus carry away whatever dirt is on the skin's surface. In cleansers, the surfactants act to remove dirt and oil, but they can also damage the top layer of the skin (the stratum corneum). When that happens, the skin's ability to hold moisture is decreased, which leads to a somewhat increased risk of contact dermatitis. In soaps the surfactants are naturally derived, but in detergents, they are artificially derived.

Soaps

"Different soaps for different folks" could be the motto of the soap industry, as any stroll through a supermarket or drug store will attest to. The soap industry has been very busy formulating all kinds of soaps for us.

It may be hard to believe, but there still are plain, old-fashioned, regular soaps, whose job it is to just help clean the skin. The cleansing agents in these soaps are ingredients such as sodium tallowate and sodium cocoate. But they also contain surfactants—sodium lauryl sulfate, cocamidopropyl betaine, and dioctyl sodium. These reduce surface tension and make the soap less abrasive when you wash.

The soap industry has developed moisturizing soaps for dry skin. These tend to have a lot of cold cream added. Surprisingly, moisturizing soaps have a lower pH than regular soaps; that is, they are *more* acidic (but not so acidic as to be irritating to the skin.)

> **Moisturizing soaps tend to have a lot of cold cream added.**

This is accomplished by adding citric or lactic acid, because these ingredients actually make the soap less irritating to the skin. Sodium laurylisethionate is another ingredient commonly present in moisturizing soaps.

Truly oily skin requires the use of a more drying type of soap. For very oily, acne-prone skin several soaps are available. Sulfur soaps, salicylic acid soaps, and benzoyl peroxide soaps can help reduce oiliness. All these are available over the counter, but the stronger benzoyl peroxide soaps are available in prescription form only.

Many people's faces have areas of oiliness and areas of normal or dry skin. This is referred to as "combination skin" and is often called "T-zone oiliness," which refers to a T-shaped area consisting of the forehead, nose, and chin. Although acne is often associated with oily skin, T-zone oiliness does not necessarily mean that you have a predisposition to acne in those areas, but you may need a stronger soap for the T-zone.

Deodorant bars are harsher than regular soaps by virtue of the addition of antibacterial ingredients such as trichlocarbon. These ingredients raise the pH of the soap, making it less acidic. Thus, the trade-off with deodorant soaps is that in order for them to fight odor effectively they generally are more irritating to the skin.

Soaps for sensitive skin are superfatted—they contain glycerin, an ingredient designed to limit how much sebum (oil) is removed from the skin.

What is the right soap for you? There is no general rule that fits for everyone, but some experts feel that the skin should stay taut for ten to fifteen minutes after you clean it, and then it should "regrease" itself. Thus, if your skin stays taut for longer than this, you may want to consider changing to a milder soap or cleanser.

If your skin stays taut longer than fifteen minutes after cleaning it, consider changing to a milder soap or cleanser.

Cleansers

Liquid cleansers come in different formulations as well. Some are soap-free. They are applied to the skin and rubbed until they foam up. Then the foam is wiped off, leaving behind a thin moisturizing film. These cleansers contain water, glycerin, cetyl alcohol, and propylene glycol.

Deodorants and Antiperspirants

Underarm odor is caused by an interaction of bacteria with sweat. Deodorants contain certain ingredients whose purpose it is to reduce the number of bacteria on the skin. Neomycin is one of the weak antibiotics often used in these products. While effective in fighting off the offending bacteria, neomycin carries with it a significant allergic potential. Other antibiotic ingredients, such as hexachlorophene, are also effective but have shown themselves to have potential toxicity, and thus they have come under stricter government regulation in recent years. Perfumes are used in deodorants to help mask body odor but have no effect upon bacteria. The only concern they might pose is an allergic reaction in people who have problems with fragrances.

Antiperspirants act by chemically preventing sweating. This is most commonly accomplished by the use of aluminum in one form or another. Although aluminum never produces an allergic reaction, its strong chemical power can irritate the skin. Aluminum can be used in different strengths. The weaker strengths are billed as being appropriate products for people with so-called delicate skin while others are billed as more "manly." Antiperspirants are often combined with deodorants to accomplish both purposes—preventing sweating *and* odor—in one product.

> **Antiperspirants act by chemically preventing sweating.**

Occasionally, other ingredients are used as antiperspirants. Some are more gentle on the skin but they are also less effective.

Adverse Reactions to Deodorants and Antiperspirants

Reactions to these deodorants and antiperspirants can range from mild to fairly extreme. Here's an example of the latter. One day when I walked into the examination room, I found a woman holding her arms up and extended, away from her body. If I didn't know better I would have thought she was preparing to fly out the window. I knew her arms had to hurt in that position, which told me that keeping them in their normal position caused her intolerable discomfort. She was pretty upset. And understandably so.

In recounting what led up to the problem, this patient said that the evening before she had used a new deodorant, then woke up with a horrendous rash in the underarm area. Since then, whenever anything, including her own skin, touched the irritated area it hurt so badly she couldn't tolerate it, which is why she had called first thing in the morning for an appointment and come right in. She was desperate to get the rash diagnosed and to get some relief. Fortunately, this skin reaction was easy to treat with a particular steroid cream, and the worst part of the irritation subsided quickly.

As with hair sprays, underarm sprays have come under fire for being potential destroyers of the ozone layer. Fortunately, roll-ons, sticks, and lotions are just as effective as long as the right ingredients are present.

Baking soda is known to absorb odors in refrigerators and is effective in the underarm area, too! Corn-

Cornstarch and baking soda are antisweat remedies.

starch is an antisweat remedy. Some people who are very sensitive to deodorants or antiperspirants have found these simple home remedies to be their saving grace.

Skin Care

Care is hard to define. Surely it includes cleanliness but goes beyond it, including the prevention of skin problems and deterioration, treatment, and even certain forms of beautification. Care products and cosmetics are generally very safe. However, due to the multitude of ingredients that go into them,

Up to 5 percent of the women who use skin care products and cosmetics will experience an adverse reaction.

some people develop problems. As a matter of fact, it has been estimated that up to 5 percent of the women who use these products will experience an adverse reaction of one sort or another during their lifetime. Although that percentage is small, when you consider the millions of women using skin care products and cosmetics in the United States, it really adds up to quite a number of people. (See below under "Cosmetics" and chapter 8.)

Astringents (Toners)

Astringents, or toners, use fragranced alcohol to remove oil from the skin. They also give a sensation of cleanliness and tightness as the alcohol dries out. Some astringents contain other ingredients, such as menthol or camphor, to induce a cool feeling. When salicylic acid or witch hazel is added to astringents, the resultant product is then considered to be an exfoliant because the extra ingredients induce light peeling, making it useful for acne-prone skin. Abrasive scrubs, cleansing masks, and mild acid agents can also cause peeling.

I see a lot of actors and actresses in my practice in the Los Angeles/Beverly Hills area. Their line of work often requires the use of heavy makeup, which can lead to pore plugging and acne formation.

I like the approach of Dr. Ellen Gendler of New York University (NYU) Medical Center who recommends a three-step makeup removal routine for actors of both sexes. Even though most of us are not professional actors, this can be useful advice for anyone who wears heavy makeup or who has a job or hobby that gets their face very dirty.

> Actresses' and actors' use of heavy makeup can lead to pore plugging and acne formation.

Step 1▸ Use a heavy cleanser to get rid of the heavy makeup.

Step 2▸ Use a light cleanser or soap to remove the residue.

Step 3▸ Use a toner, or astringent, as needed, for further touchup.

Once the skin is clean, you can reapply your everyday makeup as you desire.

Moisturizers

Moisturizers do just what the word implies—they impart moisture to the skin. The lack of moisture is the result of a decrease in the water content of the stratum corneum, which is the outermost layer of the epidermis (see chapter 2). When the skin becomes dry and flaky, moisturizers can help by one of two mechanisms: (1) they can retard or prevent water loss or (2) they can draw water into the stratum corneum.

> The skin feels dry when the water content of its outermost layer decreases—moisturizers can be of help.

The most common types of moisturizers work by preventing water loss. These are the standard commercial creams, lotions, ointments, gels, and so forth. Their formulations are varied to suit different parts of the body.

For example, most facial moisturizers are of lighter consistency, so as not to plug up pores. Daytime moisturizers are usually lotions, whereas nighttime moisturizers tend to be creams because lotions are usually more suitable cosmetically, due to their thinner consistency. Eyelid moisturizers are those same

> Hand and body moisturizers are generally thicker than their facial counterparts.

nighttime creams with some of the more irritating elements removed to avoid hurting the eye area, which is the most sensitive part of the face. Within this constellation of products can be found different products for different skin types. Oilier moisturizers cater to dry-skinned people whereas oil-free products are designed for oilier complexions.

Hand and body moisturizers are generally thicker than their facial counterparts. Creams and ointments are excellent moisturizers but can be messy, especially on areas of the body where there is hair. The discomfort many women feel from using the more greasy-feeling creams and ointments has them preferring thick lotions that spread more easily, even though these products do not moisturize as well. Hands tend to be drier than other parts of the body due to greater exposure to water, chemicals, and wind. Therefore, many hand care products, to be effective, are the thicker creams or ointments.

Some of the ingredients that are now being added to moisturizers include plant extracts, vitamins, proteins, and lipids. Although the medical literature lends only occasional support for those claims, many of my patients really feel that some of these ingredients make a difference.

A recent feature of commercial moisturizers that has received a lot of attention in the press are the liposome timed-release systems. Liposomes are microscopic moisture-releasing agents that are designed to deliver their contents to the skin for up to twelve hours. Other timed-release systems, such as microencapsulation, polymeric systems, and nanospheres have been added to the list of moisturizers as well.

The other means of moisturizing—drawing water into the stratum corneum from the humidity in the air or from the deeper layers of the epidermis—is accomplished by chemical humectants. These include glycerin, gelatin, hyaluronic acid, and propylene glycol. These can be combined with the moisturizers that prevent the skin from losing water, for a dual effect.

The latest rage in moisture research revolves around the stabilization of the skin's lipids. (Lipids are a special kind of fat.) This is based on the belief that lipids are the controlling factor in the use of water by the skin. This implies that by manipulating lipid content, the skin may be able to hold on to water more effectively.

Moisturizers of the future may also act on the life cycle of the stratum corneum by correcting defects in the formation or shedding of the inert keratin barrier that it develops. (Some "anti-aging creams" will be discussed at greater length in chapter 6.)

Sunscreens

Unlike makeup, sunscreens have been classified as drugs by the FDA. As such, they are subject to tighter regulations than substances that are classified as cosmetics even though they are over-the-counter products. This should give you a bit more peace of mind. For, these stricter regulations mean that when you buy a sunscreen you can know what you are getting. If it is marked SPF 15, it is the same strength, regardless of the price or the label.

Two types of sunscreens exist: physical agents and chemical agents. Physical agents, such as titanium dioxide or red petrolatum, act by reflecting sunlight away from the body. These are more effective than the chemical agents that operate in the ultraviolet A (UVA) range, but they are less effective than the chemical ones that operate in the ultraviolet B (UVB) spectrum of sunlight, which is where the sun's rays are strongest. In fact, most chemical sunscreens work only in the UVB range, although some newer products work in both the UVB and UVA spectrum of sunlight. Nowadays, many major brands list their protective ingredients. These sunscreens most often contain one or more of the following chemical sun blockers: para-amino benzoic acid (PABA), PABA esters, benzophenones, cinnamates, and anthrilates.

Every package of sunscreen will give the product's sun protection factor, or SPF. This is the value assigned to a sunscreen based upon its ability to protect against sunburn. If, without any sunscreen, you would ordinarily burn after ten minutes of exposure to the sun, a sunscreen with an SPF value of 6 would protect you for six times longer—you could thus go sixty minutes without burning. SPF values range from 2 to 50, but most dermatologists feel that the ones that are equal to or greater than SPF 15 will provide adequate protection for your skin.

There are elaborate charts that have been devised to "mix and match" your skin type with an SPF value to obtain your desired tan. But keep in mind the dermatologists' adage that "there is no such thing as a healthy tan." Tanned skin means burned skin, **There is no such thing as a healthy tan.** with the future potential for wrinkles, age spots, and skin cancer. The vast majority of dermatologists recommend that you stick with an SPF of 15 or above and forget about the lower numbers no matter how much you crave a tan.

Water*proof* sunscreens provide protection for up to eighty minutes of water exposure. Water-*resistant* sunscreens can protect up to forty minutes. However, both types may need to be reapplied more frequently during water exposure despite these claims.

Sunscreens come in different bases, such as gels, lotions, or creams. Waterproof sunscreens are creamier, providing better water protection but having more of a tendency to produce acne. Gels are more drying, and the alcohol content may cause stinging in the eyes.

A few sunscreen tips: Apply sunscreen about thirty minutes before you go out into the sun so that it has a chance to sink into the skin. If you are allergic to PABA, switch to a PABA-free sunscreen or a physical sunscreen. And make sure to apply enough to cover all of your exposed skin. Don't just dab it on. *Rub it in* and reapply it regularly. Remember, a single bad sunburn can significantly increase your chances of skin cancer.

> Apply sunscreen about thirty minutes before you go out into the sun.

A final word. A few years ago an article appeared in a major dermatology journal that raised a few eyebrows across the country. It reported on research into sunscreen use in elderly people. The study showed that sunscreens might block sunlight so effectively that vitamin D, which needs sunlight to activate it in the skin, would not be produced. Since vitamin D is essential to calcium metabolism and thus to bone strength, and with osteoporosis already a major problem in the elderly, the authors felt that sunscreen use could actually be harmful to this age group by interfering with their ability to get the vitamin D from the sun. But most experts feel that the benefits of sunscreen use far outweigh any of their suspected disadvantages for any age group.

Home Remedies, Natural Products, Over-the-Counter Preparations

Unlike the other organs of the body, the skin is directly exposed to the rough and tumble of everyday life. As a result, it suffers lots of comparatively minor and occasionally major assaults in the forms of bruises, burns, scrapes, and infections. Depending on their degree of seriousness, these do not always need to be treated with a fancy prescription. Many "balms" can be purchased without a prescription in drug stores or health food stores, or can even be concocted from products found in your own home.

Although these remedies are often effective, they can't cure everything. And, like the more potent prescription medicines, they can have side effects. The best example of this is with the oral preparation aspirin. Each year a certain number of people die as a result of aspirin sensitivity. Excessive use of over-the-counter drugs such as acetaminophen (Tylenol) can lead to liver toxicity or death.

So keep in mind when you read this section that over-the-counter preparations, natural products, and home remedies don't always work and, on occasion, can actually hurt you. When using these preparations, use good judgment. Abandon them at the first indication of a bad reaction. And if in a reasonable period of time they don't remedy the problem for which you are using them, don't postpone seeking professional medical advice.

The Naturals

Many centuries ago, Cleopatra is said to have used a special mixture of herbs to keep her skin looking youthful. Romantic tales of her beauty sent many a person in search of the magic formula that she used. Although the history and full evaluation of the natural products being used and sold as skin remedies is beyond the scope of this book, aloe vera is one I want to talk about because it has received some serious attention in dermatological circles.

Is there any rational pharmacologic reason why the juice of the aloe vera plant should work? Yes, says Allen J. Natow, M.D., of the New York University Medical Center in New York City. At least four different active ingredients have been identified in aloe compounds. Two of them act against bradykinin and prostaglandin. Bradykinin is the substance responsible for pain at sites of inflammation. Prostaglandin, so named because it was first isolated from the prostate gland (but is present in both males and females), is an important mediator of inflammation. By blocking bradykinin and prostaglandin, aloe vera helps decrease the pain and inflammation associated with rashes and skin ulcers. Another special property of aloe vera is its ability to act as a humectant—it helps keep water in the skin. Because of that, it is frequently used in cosmetics as a skin moisturizer and smoother.

> At least four different active ingredients have been identified in aloe compounds.

Not that aloe vera is a foolproof substance. As with any other plant, allergic reactions to it can develop. It's ironic that aloe vera, which can be used to treat plant allergies, can itself cause them. Aloe vera is part of a trend towards natural products. Its use has spurred interest within the scientific community to have a new look at some old substances for their effectiveness in care and treatment.

There are quite a few herbs that certain of the holistic health people find to have a salutary effect. Although the field of alternative medicine raises much controversy within traditional medical circles, its practitioners claim to help many skin problems with their methods.

If you experiment with herbal or other natural remedies, follow the same precautions you'd use with any home remedy or over-the-counter medication—use as little as possible, and stop if the problem gets worse.

Home Remedies

Drug and health food stores aren't the only sources of effective remedies. Some can be found on the shelves in your own kitchen or from the water that comes from your tap. For example, cold compresses or cool baths will help bring some relief to itchy skin conditions like poison ivy, poison oak, insect bites, chicken pox, or eczema. Oatmeal may be added to the bath water for a soothing effect. Dr. Abigail Givens, Chief of Dermatology at Children's Hospital in Oakland, California, recommends that you cook the oatmeal first and then dissolve it in the bath water. Baking soda in cool bath water is also helpful, according to Dr. Givens.

Applying a cream, lotion, or ointment to the skin right after a bath locks in moisture. However, if the lotion has an alcohol, or even a water, base, it can cause a burning sensation when applied to broken skin. Ointments are less likely to irritate the skin.

Should small cuts be covered with a bandage or left open to breathe? There is considerable debate over this seemingly small matter. Both approaches have their pros and cons. If a wound is on an exposed area, where it is likely to get contaminated with germs or dirt, it is probably better to keep it covered.

Soothe and clean a burn by running cold water over it.

Is there any truth that putting butter on a burn makes it heal better? There is nothing in butter itself that leads to better wound healing. It is the coldness of an applied substance that helps to soothe and dissipate some of the heat from the burn. In that regard, any cold substance will suffice. Running cold tap water over a burn is often suggested. It cools and cleans at the same time.

Over-the-Counter Preparations

There are over-the-counter preparations (sometimes referred to as OTCs) for an enormous number of problems, as any visit to a drug store or supermarket amply demonstrates. What follows is a discussion of some of the categories of these products that are most frequently used for skin care.

Antibacterials

Topical antibacterials are used to fight the germs that cause infection in superficial wounds, cuts, and burns. Many require no prescription. The most frequently used antibiotic in these preparations is neomycin. Some have just one antibiotic in them, while others have several. Iodine ointments and solutions also have an antibacterial effect, although they tend to sting and stain. Mercury-containing compounds, like mercurochrome, used to be one of the mainstays of topical antibacterial treatment, but they have given way in recent years to products that are less irritating.

Wound Healing

Zinc has been used since antiquity to promote wound healing, and zinc-containing ointments are still in use for this purpose. They are good for diaper rash; however, because they are opaque they are shunned for facial use.

Pain Relief

Pain relief remedies are always in demand. The "caine" family of topical anesthetics includes benzocaine, lidocaine, and mepyrlycaine. These act by temporarily numbing the local nerve endings. Be careful, though. Benzocaine, a common ingredient in over-the-counter ointments for pain, is a frequent cause of allergic reactions. Because it is a PABA derivative, and PABA is the most common ingredient in sunscreens, people who become allergic to benzocaine may cross-react with PABA-containing sunscreens and then develop an allergic

> Benzocaine, a common ingredient in over-the-counter ointments for pain, is a frequent cause of allergic reactions.

reaction to these sunscreens. Likewise, people with allergic reactions to PABA sunscreens should stay away from benzocaine.

Itching Relief

Menthol is helpful with itching. It comes in the form of creams, soaps, shampoos, and other products. The mentholated patches that are popular for aches and pains are helpful for itchy skin as well. Camphor and phenol are two other ingredients that have anti-itch and somewhat anesthetic (pain- or sensation-killing) properties. Topical antihistamines may also afford some relief for itching, but they are not as effective as oral antihistamine preparations.

Acne Care

Acne products make up a large share of the topical skin care market. Benzoyl peroxide compounds are big sellers. As with hydrogen peroxide, benzoyl peroxide has drying and antibacterial properties. Thus it serves as a good acne remedy by drying up lesions and fighting off the bacteria in those lesions. The higher, prescription strengths are more drying but may be quite irritating.

Acne products work by drying up the skin and fighting bacteria in the acne.

Astringent lotions and soaps also serve to dry out acne and the excessive oil that often accompanies it. Abrasive bars and sponges may improve some of the plugged up pores and help remove dead cells from the skin surface. They should be used with caution, however, so as not to irritate the skin.

Steroids for Itching and Inflammation

Hydrocortisone creams and lotions used to be prescription-only products. Then, several years ago the FDA allowed .5 percent (½ percent) hydrocortisone to be sold without a prescription. Most recently, 1 percent hydrocortisone has joined the over-the-counter ranks.

When applied topically, hydrocortisone has a good anti-itch action. The potential side effect of stronger prescription strength topical cortisone products is that with prolonged and excessive use, they can thin out the skin permanently. This can result in wrinkling and in the skin looking red, because the underlying blood vessels show through the thinned-out skin. One percent hydrocortisone is generally safe in this regard, but like the stronger prescription creams and ointments, it should be used with caution on the facial and genital areas because the skin in these areas of the body is thinner. When using over-the-counter topical steroids don't exceed the recommended dosage strength or the length of treatment recommended on the package. And never use stronger prescription strength topical steroids without medical supervision.

The anti-inflammatory action of *oral* cortisone products makes them helpful in arthritis, autoimmune diseases, and skin irritations, among other conditions.

Are cortisone products bad for you? Not if you follow your physician's directions for their use and, in the case of the over-the-counter cortisone topicals, you follow the directions on the package. Cortisone is no exception to the rule that any drug can be bad for you if used improperly.

People sometimes hesitate to use cortisone—a *catabolic* steroid—because they confuse it with a different class of steroids— the *anabolic* steroids—which are controversial because of their use (and abuse) by body builders and other athletes. The anabolic steroids have a number of unhealthy side effects, which are compounded when they are used in high doses.

Cortisone, although a steroid, acts differently than the anabolic steroids do. It breaks down the inflammatory enzymes that cause rashes or itching (and it also helps in other inflammatory conditions, like some forms of arthritis). When used properly it can often bring considerable relief. The anabolic steroids act to increase body and muscle bulk.

Cosmetics

Most people suspect, and are thus not surprised to learn, that the cosmetics industry is one of the largest consumer-driven industries in the country. More money is spent annually on cosmetics than on prescription drugs.

Some cosmetics are regulated by the FDA and some are not. The distinction between what is considered a *cosmetic drug* and what is considered just a *cosmetic* is the subject of hot governmental debate. The FDA defines a cosmetic drug as something that "changes the structures and functions of the skin." The result of this distinction means that toothpaste, antiperspirants, and sunscreens are considered cosmetic drugs whereas makeup is not.

This has a major implication in the world of nonprescription drugs. Cosmetic drugs are subject to stricter regulations than makeup. Thus, certain claims can be made about them that cannot be made about nondrug cosmetics (like makeup). For example, toothpaste can claim to make your teeth whiter. Makeup cannot claim to *make* your skin younger, but it can purport to make it *look* younger. The former ("make") implies that the product can actually achieve a physical change; the latter ("look") implies only the *appearance* of change. In terms of actual impact on potential customers, however, this difference may be insignificant. But another impact of this categorization is that since makeup is not considered a drug, it has fewer restrictions than the cosmetics that are considered drugs.

Cosmetic companies must, however, demonstrate the safety of their products, whether or not they are considered drugs. This is no small matter, especially in light of a recent report in the *Journal of Clinical Pharmacy and Therapeutics* about bacterial contamination of foreign cosmetics. A study in Egypt and Jordan found heavy bacterial contamination in 4 percent of the eye shadows tested, 5 percent of the face creams tested, and 15 percent of the mascaras tested. Fungal contamination was also quite prevalent. Imagine rubbing a handful of bacteria and fungus on your face every time you put on makeup! The FDA tries hard to prevent such situations in this country.

Despite the close regulation of the cosmetic industry, however, there are still some gray areas regarding labeling of products. Watch out for so-called oil-free cosmetics. Although they may be free of natural oils—like mineral oil—these cosmetics may contain synthetic oils, which also can cause acne.

> The so-called oil-free cosmetics may contain synthetic oils, which also can cause acne.

You should also watch out for cosmetics that are labeled "fragrance-free." Even if the product has no scent or odor, it may contain masking fragrances. These serve to block the odor of other ingredients in order to achieve a neutral "nonsmell." So, when products have no noticeable odor or even when they are marked "unscented" or "fragrance-free," given current regulations, they may still contain added fragrances. This is important to know because fragrance is the most common cause of allergic skin reactions to cosmetics.

Facial Cosmetics

Lipstick

The basic ingredients of lipstick are wax and oil mixed together. Other ingredients are then added to give color, texture, flavor, and/or scent. Interestingly, although ingredients are sometimes added to prevent chapping from wind and cold, the lipstick itself may cause an allergy, which itself can cause chapping. Some lipsticks contain sunscreen to prevent fever blisters or burning. PABA is often used for this purpose, so people who are allergic to it should be aware of its possible presence in some lipsticks. Even though lipstick covers the lips, sometimes it can actually make you more sensitive to the sun. The combination of lipstick and sun exposure can cause a rash, which is most often a reaction to the dye in the lipstick. Lanolin, a widely used softening agent in lipstick, may also be a source of allergy. Fortunately, the lips are a fairly resistant part of the body. Allergic reactions are usually mild and quickly disappear when the product is discontinued. As with the other classes of skin care products, hypoallergenic lipstick may be of help to sensitive persons.

Caution should always be exercised in sharing lipstick or lip balm with someone who has active herpes infection of the lips ("cold sores" or "fever blisters") because the virus is contagious.

Foundations, Powder, Rouge, and Blush

Foundations are available not only in different shades but also for different skin types: dry, oily, or normal. Powders may be either loose or pressed. Rouges and blushes, which are only applied to a small area of the face, where foundation and powder have often already been applied, don't really need to vary with skin type.

Allergic reactions to these facial products are rare. But, foundations and powders, which are applied to those parts of the face that are acne-prone, can cause acne. Products that cause acne are called comedogenic. This is because they plug up the pores and cause whiteheads and blackheads, or comedones.

> **Foundations and powders can cause acne, so use products labeled as "noncomedogenic."**

Oil-based makeup is the most likely to be comedogenic. Other ingredients, such as cocoa butter or oleic acid, are known acne producers, too. Lighter creams, made with no oil, are preferable for acne-prone individuals. In general, foundations with a matte or nonshiny appearance are oil-free and have the least comedogenic potential.

To be labeled noncomedogenic a product must pass a test performed on a rabbit's ear to see whether or not it produces acne. Although a rabbit's ear may seem a far cry from a woman's face, it does work well to test cosmetics for their comedogenic potential on women's facial skin. It is an accepted way to determine if a substance does or doesn't produce acne.

Shinier foundations are better moisturizers. They have an oilier consistency, so they are popular among women with dry skin.

Shinier foundations are better moisturizers.

These also wear longer than matte or semi-matte foundations.

Some foundations have been combined with sunscreens, meaning that you don't have to forgo your cosmetics to have sun protection. But there are some experts who feel that these combination products are neither good foundations nor good sunscreens. They recommend using separate products, one for each purpose.

Dr. Beverly Johnson of Howard University Medical Center in Washington, D.C., has pointed out that African Americans may have a particular problem finding the right cosmetic due to their wider range of skin shades. Another concern with facial cosmetics for African American women is related to their propensity to develop postinflammatory hyperpigmentation (dark spots in response to pimples—see chapter 8). This makes foundation coverage difficult because any irritation can potentially lead to postinflammatory hyperpigmentation. To reduce the chances of irritation and acne, Dr. Johnson recommends fragrance-free makeup for African American women.

Eye Makeup

The eyelids are perhaps the most sensitive part of the body's surface. The area is very thin in comparison with other parts of the skin and, as such, is easily irritated. Smoke, dust, and wind are just some of the elements that can bother the eyes as well as the skin around them.

Cosmetics manufacturers are acutely aware of the sensitive nature of the eyelids. They take every precaution in preparing their products so that problems will not occur. The FDA has placed eye care products and makeup in a special cate-

The FDA has placed eye care products and makeup in a special category.

gory. Paraphenylene-diamine, the backbone of hair dyes, is prohibited in products applied to areas near the eyes. Similarly, only certain colors, which are insoluble in water, are FDA approved for eye makeup.

Eye shadow comes in a variety of types. Greasy ointments, smooth creams, lotions, or powders are available. Each has a different chemical composition. In general, allergic reactions are uncommon, but caution should be used if any irritation is experienced.

Eyeliners also come in several forms. The pencil type is similar to eyebrow pencil and should be used carefully so as not to scratch the eyeball. Liquid eyeliners can smudge onto the eyeball.

Over the last few years, a process known as permanent eyeliner has been developed. This involves tattooing pigment onto the edges of the eyelids so that the color is permanent. It was originally devised for women with arthritis who have trouble applying their eye liner. Unfortunately, an occasional allergic reaction to the tattoo pigment will occur, which, as you can imagine, presents a major problem—how to remove the tattoo material without disfiguring the eyelid.

Mascara is seldom a problem in terms of allergy. However, when it runs or smears, it

Allergic reactions with mascara and artificial eyelashes are rare.

can annoy or irritate the eye. Artificial eyelashes are relatively problem free.

Other Cosmetics

We've just looked at most of the products used to enhance the appearance of your face. Here are some other products used, also with attractiveness in mind but for other parts of the body as well or to appeal to our sense of smell.

Perfume

Fragrances are available as perfumes—purely for the purpose of helping you achieve a desired body scent—or as ingredients in commercial skin care products and cosmetics.

Thousands of perfumes are available on the market today. Their major components are aromatic chemicals. Usually these are synthetic compounds, but animal or plant extracts are also used.

Perfumes can produce any one of the three basic adverse reactions—allergy, irritation, or photosensitivity (see chapter 8). Skin eruptions are, however, usually mild. A specific photosensitive reaction known as *berloque dermatitis* may produce a dark pigmentation of the skin that can last for months. An allergic response may also result in the form of hives.

Bronzing Gels and Tanning Lotions

Bronzing gels and tanning lotions are another category of product about which there is some controversy and confusion. Despite the brown color they impart to the skin, these products generally do not provide sun protection; they merely stain the skin surface. There are some that do contain a built-in sunscreen, but these products offer only temporary protection. A helpful hint regarding tanning lotions is that they must be applied quickly and evenly to avoid streaking. Also, make sure to wash your hands right away after application so that the palms of your hands don't tan.

> **Bronzing gels do not provide sun protection—they merely stain the skin surface.**

Skin Bleaches

Preparations used to lighten or bleach the skin in order to get rid of freckles or lentigines (liver spots) most usually contain an ingredient known as hydroquinone. A 2 percent concentration is available in over-the-counter skin bleaches, while a 3 or 4 percent concentration is available by prescription only.

> **Lemon juice really can bleach freckles and liver spots—but can irritate the skin.**

As one might expect, bleaching agents can irritate the skin, especially the ones that are prescription strength, which are stronger. Allergic reactions are possible as well. A common complaint with some of the greasier bleaching creams—sometimes called fade creams—is that they tend to aggravate acne. Bleaching creams that use active ingredients other than hydroquinones are available also, but they have the same basic potential for side effects.

A time-honored bleaching remedy is citrus fruit juice, especially lemon juice. To a certain degree, it really works. Sometimes, however, because of its acidity, it too can irritate the skin.

Chapter 6

Medical and Surgical Approaches to Cosmetic Problems

....

Wrinkles, age spots, tattoos, baggy eyelids, and acne scarring—these are just
a few of the cosmetic problems that makeup is not very successful
in covering. Even where it does work, it takes a good bit of skill,
patience, and time every single day. So, people have looked to the
field of medicine for more effective, longer lasting cosmetic remedies. Physicians and pharmacologists have responded to this quest
with treatments and surgical procedures that offer a real measure
of cosmetic success.

This chapter starts with a discussion of topical cosmetic treatments—the creams, ointments, lotions, and gels you apply directly
to the skin. The emphasis is on Retin-A and the alpha-hydroxy-
acids (AHAs) because these are the most medically respected and
popular of the topical cosmetic treatments.

I'll give some of the history of how each was developed—
these are particularly interesting stories and ones that shed light on
the nature of the drugs themselves—plus a close look at the cosmetic conditions that Retin-A and the AHAs benefit, the rules for
their use, their side effects, and how they compare. Then, I review
some of the "wonder" creams that we were led to believe would do
marvelous things for the skin but that ultimately fell far short of
their claims and expectations.

Next, I discuss the main techniques and procedures used for cosmetic treatment for a wide range of conditions—collagen injections, chemical peels, dermabrasion, the face lift, and liposuction.

Immediately following that comes a section on the different kinds of cosmetic problems people bring to physicians to "fix"— problems like torn earlobes, tattoos, baggy eyelids, excess fat, and more. Here, I give you an idea of the challenges each of these problems presents to the doctor, what the patient will likely experience from these treatments, what precautions should be taken, any associated discomforts, side effects, and, most importantly, what can be reasonably expected in terms of results or outcomes. You'll find descriptions of techniques and procedures—like blepharoplasty for baggy eyelids or laser removal of tattoos—that are specific to particular cosmetic problems. Each discussion in this section ends with a list of the questions most frequently asked about these problems and their remedies, along with their answers.

The chapter ends with a bit of a question and answer free-for-all about all sorts of cosmetic concerns and treatments.

Although in my private practice of dermatology, I use many of the treatments and procedures discussed in this chapter, my comments here should not be treated as advocacy. Just as with everything else in this book, my aim is to provide a balanced, sober, fair discussion so that you can get a comprehensive and sound picture of what this field of medical practice is about, what it can offer, and what its limitations are.

I would be remiss if, in discussing cosmetic medicine and surgery, I failed to point out that attitudes toward this field of medical practice are quite mixed. Our society is ambivalent about using medical resources to deal with matters of appearance. So, almost everyone who chooses to have cosmetic treatment has to pay out of their own pockets.

Nevertheless, it is not just the wealthiest people in the country who get cosmetic treatment. Lots of ordinary people do. Last year, there were hundreds of thousands of cosmetic procedures performed in the United States. The majority of them were on women. Cosmetic treatment is big business, with millions of dollars spent annually by consumers, manufacturers, physicians, and hospitals.

I'll leave it to others to debate the issue of who gets cosmetic treatment, why they do, how society regards it, and whether medical insurance should pay for it.

As a dermatologist, my purpose here is very specific. I want to share with you as much as I can about cosmetic medical and surgical treatment. This area of medical practice is one that abounds in myths but not in accurate public information. This is especially critical because most of us are particularly vulnerable to claims about improving our physical appeal and making ourselves into more perfect specimens. That vulnerability combined with an absence of sound information can often prevent us from acting in our own rational self-interest. So, for the sake of your health, your appearance, and even your pocketbook, it is vital to sort through the promotional promises and frequently inaccurate, thirdhand, word-of-mouth stories.

However, if you are seriously considering getting medical help with a cosmetic problem, no book can substitute for the information that will emerge from a discussion with a physician you respect. This is especially true in so personal and subjective a matter as cosmetic surgery. To help you get the most out of your interaction with your physician, you might want to first do a little research on your own, then discuss the following sorts of questions and any others you might have with your doctor.

1▶ What do you expect cosmetic surgery will be able to achieve for you?
2▶ What are the true potential benefits?
3▶ What are the risks?
4▶ In the case of larger surgeries, are you ready for the physical and psychological impact of the trauma as well as the change in your appearance? (Sometimes people are unhappy with a certain aspect of their appearance but can't easily accept the change involved in its remedy.)
5▶ How long will the results last?
6▶ Is there variation in success rates at different medical institutions and with different doctors?

But even with the most careful investigation, not every question can be resolved. As is the case in most every area of medicine, there are still many unanswered questions regarding the hows and whys of cosmetic prescription creams and surgery. How safe is safe? Are there some undesirable side effects that still haven't been recognized? Might a better approach to any particular cosmetic problem be in the works, meaning that maybe you should wait? These are not easy questions to answer. But, as with other important decisions in life, we often make them with less than complete or perfect information. We simply try to get the best information available. If we feel it's solid enough, we then use it to balance risk against benefit and then proceed. Hence, this chapter.

Topical Preparations for Cosmetic Treatment

For centuries, creams and ointments have been advertised as being capable of erasing wrinkles, age spots, and other signs of aging. It is only recently that we have begun to see topical preparations that provide a strong scientific basis for such claims. Retin-A was the first to come to medical and general public notice.

The Retin-A Story

Its announcement, its history, what it does, questions and controversies, and then some.

The News Conference

On a cool New York City day in January of 1988, in the prestigious Rainbow Room at Rockefeller Center, a major announcement was about to be made. John Voorhees, M.D., chairman of the Department of Dermatology at the University of Michigan, stepped up to the microphone. Voorhees had gained fame in dermatology circles mostly for his work on the common skin disorder psoriasis. But this day was different. He and his co-workers had been working on what was reported to be the definitive study of Retin-A. At this momentous occasion in Rockefeller Center, when the results were about to be announced, the world stood up and took notice.

The study was very basic but incredibly revealing. Forty people (all volunteers) with sun-damaged skin were given two tubes of cream. One contained a placebo, that is, an inert substance with no biologic effect. The other contained Retin-A, a cream known for its beneficial effect on acne. Half of the participants rubbed the placebo cream on their face and left forearm and rubbed the Retin-A on their right forearm. The other half did the reverse. The study employed one of the most respected research designs in science—the double blind design. In such a study participants and researchers alike do not know who is getting the treatment and who, the placebo. This allows the results of the study to be free from any bias that could result had they known which was which. Results from such studies can't be interpreted (and dismissed) as being self-fulfilling prophecies.

So, without knowing which was which, the participants faithfully used the two creams each night for four months. Of the forty who began the study, ten dropped out for various personal or medical reasons, leaving thirty participants remaining. That represents a dropout rate that is well within the boundaries of what is to be expected in studies like this.

The results of the study revealed that fourteen out of the fifteen people who used Retin-A on their faces showed improvement in their sun-damaged skin, while *none* of those using the placebo got better. Not only that, but all thirty participants showed improvement on the forearm to which Retin-A had been applied, while none showed improvement on their placebo-treated forearm. Amazing results! At first it seemed almost unbelievable, as reflected in the saying, "If something *seems* too good to be true, it probably *is* too good to be true."

But the Voorhees group had come prepared with detailed analyses to back up their results. It was clear that they had put considerable effort into making their study scientifically sound. First, all of the participants were evaluated by the same doctor so that the results weren't affected by variations between evaluators. All participants were evaluated for the *type* of improvement they experienced. Improvement in fine wrinkling headed the list. Skin hue, coarse wrinkling, and roughness were also found to be helped. The *degree* of improvement each participant experienced was rated using three categories: (1) much improved, (2) improved, and (3) slightly improved. The results of this evaluation of facial skin revealed that one person was considered to be "much improved," ten were "improved," and three were "slightly improved." In short, the skin treated with Retin-A looked and felt smoother and less wrinkled.

Let's face it, though. As objective as one tries to be, personal prejudice may creep into the evaluation of what is considered improved and what is not. What about some solid data that leaves no room for argument? The Voorhees group had thought of that as well. That's why, both before and after the Retin-A was used, small pieces of skin (biopsies) were taken from each of the thirty people who participated. These were analyzed under the microscope.

The results of the biopsies supported the evidence that had been reported on the basis of the examinations done with the naked eye. The microscopic analysis demonstrated that the very top part of the skin, the stratum corneum, which governs the roughness of the skin, had been made much thinner and more compact by the Retin-A. That made the skin look and feel smoother. The epidermis—the layer of skin that lies just beneath the stratum corneum—changed also, but it became thicker. In fact, the epidermal layer of the Retin-A treated areas increased a whopping 273 percent in thickness, while the placebo-treated areas increased in thickness by only 18 percent. This meant that the skin treated with Retin-A that had previously been thin and wrinkled had become thicker, smoother, and less wrinkled. The Retin-A also turned off the melanocytes, the pigment-producing cells of the skin that lie at the bottom of the epidermis. This had the effect of diminishing the color of the age spots.

> **Retin-A makes the skin look and feel smoother.**

What was perhaps most impressive to dermatologists was the effect of Retin-A on the dermis—the layer of skin that lies underneath the epidermis. There had been widespread skepticism about Retin-A's ability to effectively penetrate into the deeper layers of the skin. However, the biopsies showed that the blood vessels in the dermis were widened and were carrying more blood to the skin. This accounted for the skin's rosy color that 75 percent of the participants reported noting.

It certainly appeared that, finally, a wonder cream had lived up to its promise.

Dr. Voorhees and his colleagues also spoke of some problems with Retin-A. Almost all of the participants—92 percent of them—experienced some degree of rash from using the cream, although only 8 percent of the total number who participated withdrew as a result. Some who did develop the rash experienced it for up to three months, while others seemed to acclimate to Retin-A after a few weeks, meaning the rash went away. A moisturizing cream proved helpful with the rash, but almost one-third of the participants required a potent topical steroid (cortisone) cream to relieve it.

The Discovery of Retin-A

As with most discoveries, Retin-A did not just appear overnight. The person generally acknowledged to be its discoverer is Albert Kligman, M.D. Flamboyant and flashy, he was, at the time, the chairman of the Department of Dermatology at the University of Pennsylvania. In addition to his medical degree, Dr. Kligman possesses a Ph.D. in botany. In the early 1960s, armed with considerable vision and with a deep interest in understanding the fundamentals of how human skin functions, he began studying Retin-A.

Among the numerous scientific articles he published on Retin-A's effects was one published in October 1986. This was fifteen months before the dramatic announcement of Dr. Voorhees. Writing in the *Journal of the American Academy of Dermatology*, Kligman reported on a study in which he evaluated more than four hundred women between the ages of forty-eight and sixty-five, all of whom used Retin-A once a day for at least six months. In contrast to the Voorhees study announced two years later, Kligman's reported that the visible changes on the forearm after three months of Retin-A use were rather slight—there was only some decrease in roughness. The effect of Retin-A on the face was a different matter. He found it to be more impressive than on the forearm, which was confirmed by the Voorhees study. Kligman also noted that the most damaged skin showed the greatest improvement.

Another important fact that came to light from the Kligman study was that with Retin-A, microscopic actinic keratoses were eliminated from the skin. These are precancerous growths that are very common in sun-damaged skin (see chapters 3 and 8). If left untreated, these can go on to develop into squamous cell carcinomas, a deadly type of skin cancer. So, Retin-A's beneficial effects were found to be not just cosmetic but therapeutic as well.

> Retin-A eliminates microscopic actinic keratoses—the precancerous growths that are very common in sun-damaged skin.

Kligman, like Voorhees after him, did extensive skin biopsies as part of his study. In fact, much of what Voorhees had done and found had already been accomplished by Kligman. This also included finding that Retin-A penetrated into the dermis (the second layer of the skin) to cause the formation of new collagen, the fiber that gives the skin its strength. This occurred on the face but not on the forearm, which probably explains why he found that the improvement on the forearm was not as impressive as it was on the face.

Yet Voorhees and Kligman did not agree on everything. Kligman reported that sun-induced age spots (lentigines) were unresponsive to Retin-A treatment, although he did concede that they may lighten somewhat. Voorhees, on the other hand, came out with a much bolder claim. He concluded that the majority of age spots *did* improve with Retin-A therapy.

Why did Dr. Voorhees's study make so much larger a splash than Dr. Kligman's of only less than a year and a half earlier—especially since it was Dr. Kligman who developed Retin-A and found very much the same things in his study that Dr. Voorhees found in his?

Both studies were published in prestigious medical journals. The Voorhees study appeared in the *Journal of the American Medical Association* and Kligman's appeared in the *Journal of the American Academy of Dermatology*. But although both journals are prestigious, these two publications have a very different readership and circulation. The one Kligman published in—the *Journal of the American Academy of Dermatology*—is directed solely to dermatologists, with a circulation of roughly ten thousand. The *Journal of the American Medical Association*, where the Voorhees study was published, covers a very wide range of topics in medicine and, at the time, had a readership of several hundred thousand. It is read by general internists, family practice physicians, and physicians from a wide range of medical specialties. And because of the scope of medical issues it covers, the *Journal of the American Medical Association* is more likely to come to the attention of the press, which is always looking for medical news, especially exciting breakthroughs in medicine.

But other factors influenced the different level of interest and attention these two studies attracted. The Voorhees study was considered by some to be more scientific than the Kligman study since it used a double blind experimental design (described above), while Kligman's study did not.

Even more important, the Voorhees article contained before-and-after color photographs of the participants, while Kligman's contained none. There is considerable truth in the clichés "seeing is believing," and "one picture is worth a thousand words." That's why those photos were so important. However, what was really critical in getting dermatologists from all over North America to begin prescribing Retin-A for their patients was that *two* independent studies, conducted by *two* of the *top* dermatologists in the country, reported out such striking results and *agreed* on so many points. While all the hoopla came with the Voorhees announcement, the fact that the two very respected studies validated each other was what really packed the punch.

Dermatologists then found that their clinical experience confirmed what the studies had reported: Retin-A *did* help undo some of the damage the sun had done to their patients' skin. The popularity of Retin-A is very obvious from its sales figures. In 1991, its manufacturer, Ortho Pharmaceuticals, sold over $100 million worth of Retin-A cream.

However, Retin-A does have its critics. Some dermatologists will prescribe it only for acne, preferring to wait and see whether the newer claims for improvement in wrinkles and age spots hold up. Others worry about prescribing so powerful a drug for primarily cosmetic reasons, due to its potential for skin irritation.

There are also some suspicions that Retin-A's popularity may simply be the result of Ortho's skill at public relations. The television program "60 Minutes," on February 4, 1990, showed that some of the purportedly independent dermatologists who praised Retin-A were in fact paid by the manufacturer. This cast a shadow on the credibility of the praise being put forth for this product.

Many of these questions and concerns have been resolved as dermatologists and patients have accumulated experience with the drug. Also, in the time that has passed since the original studies were done, newer studies, all done with respectable scientific methodology and independent of Ortho, have supported the work of Voorhees and Kligman. These have put the credibility question raised by the "60 Minutes" piece to rest. However, despite the quality of the scientific studies done with Retin-A, some controversy remains, partly because it is new and partly because careful clinicians are conservative about jumping on the bandwagon of new treatments. They know all too well that it takes a good while before all the effects of a drug are known.

From Vitamin A to Retin-A

The Retin-A story goes back many years, beginning with vitamin A. Like most of the other vitamins, vitamin A was discovered early in this century. The chemical name for vitamin A is *retinol* and, like Retin-A, the name of practically every substance derived from it reflects that name. Vitamin A was called retinol because scientists observed a connection between vitamin A and the health and functioning of the eye, specifically the retina. Deficiencies in vitamin A resulted in visual problems involving the retina.

The relationship between vitamin A and good eyesight is reflected in the well-known saying, "You never saw a rabbit wearing glasses." But, joking aside, vitamin A is essential not only to maintaining baseline vision but to healthy skin as well. A vitamin A deficiency will cause dry, red skin with thick flakes.

It was around 1932 that it was realized that the administration of high doses of vitamin A would cut down on the scaliness of the skin. This led to the use of high-dose vitamin A in the treatment of psoriasis, a skin condition characterized by thick, white scales that can occur on the elbows, knees, scalp, or anywhere else on the body. The high-dose vitamin A treatment worked somewhat for psoriasis but, unfortunately, it introduced a new medical problem that had not been known about before. In the higher doses like those necessary to treat psoriasis, vitamin A can produce symptoms of headache, ringing in the ears, hair loss, and, if continued for long periods of time, liver damage. So, for an effective psoriasis treatment, it was back to the drawing board.

With the twin revelations that, on the one hand, vitamin A helped the skin quite remarkably but, on the other, when taken orally in the large doses needed to achieve those results, it caused unacceptable side effects, researchers began wondering whether they could find a way to deliver this vitamin directly to the skin via a *topical* preparation. But when they tried it, they had no luck. It had absolutely no effect upon the skin.

Most investigators stopped right there. But G. Stuttgen, Ph.D., took it a step further. In wondering why vitamin A worked for dry skin when taken by mouth but not when applied topically to the skin, he thought perhaps it was not the vitamin A that was effective but, instead, one of its breakdown products. (A breakdown product is something produced as a result of certain enzymes or other biochemicals working on a substance—in this case vitamin A—inside the body.) This led him to do research on one of the major breakdown products of vitamin A—a substance called tretinoin.

Dr. Stuttgen's studies revealed that the first effects of applying tretinoin (the chemical name for Retin-A) to the skin were redness and irritation. However, he noticed that after a bit of time passed, there was a dramatic improvement in a skin condition known as ichthyosis, or "alligator skin," which afflicts many people. This condition is characterized by thick, dry, brown scales that adhere to the skin's surface. The improvement brought about by tretinoin was very much in keeping with the success achieved when oral vitamin A

Tretinoin was the first non-toxic treatment capable of flattening and removing the scales associated with ichthyosis ("alligator skin").

had been used (in the earlier days) for psoriasis, a condition whose symptoms are very much like those of ichthyosis. But even though tretinoin was the first non-toxic treatment capable of flattening and removing the scales associated with ichthyosis, it did not gain wide acceptance because it produced redness and irritation. So, even though it was effective and wasn't found to be toxic (as oral vitamin A had been), its side effects kept it from being adopted as a substitute treatment.

Nothing much happened with tretinoin until the late 1960s when Dr. Kligman began accumulating scientific evidence that Retin-A was an effective treatment for acne. Kligman showed that tretinoin, which came to be called Retin-A, worked by increasing the rate of skin turnover, thereby causing the skin to eliminate blackheads and whiteheads.

In the late 1960s, scientific evidence emerged to show that Retin-A was an effective treatment for acne.

As interest grew, more investigators jumped on the bandwagon, including Dr. Voorhees. By 1975, the first international conference on Retin-A was held, and scientists shared their knowledge of how and why Retin-A worked on the skin.

Interestingly, the success of this *topical* vitamin A derivative sparked research into a search for an *oral* derivative that would be effective but not have the toxic side effects of oral vitamin A. Out of this effort, in the early 70s, the oral retinoids were introduced. Like oral vitamin A, the first studies showed these vitamin A derivatives to be very effective *but* very toxic. Eventually, a seemingly safer and effective related compound, known as *isotretinoin*, was developed. It was marketed under the name brand name Accutane, and it has proved to be a powerful drug for the treatment of severe acne. When it was released for use in the early 1980s, it seemed to be the savior for people with previously resistant cystic acne.

It is recommended that women of childbearing age should make sure to use the most effective methods of birth control while they are taking Accutane.

However, problems emerged. In fact, Accutane was later almost withdrawn from the market forever when pregnant women who took the drug gave birth to severely malformed babies. Instead of withdrawing it, however, the FDA forced its manufacturer to engage in extensive doctor and patient education programs concerning its danger in pregnancy. It is recommended that women of childbearing age should make sure to use the most effective methods of birth control while they are taking Accutane.

Retin-A: Its Practical Applications and Limits

As Retin-A has been worked with, both at the research and clinical level, it has emerged as useful in the treatment of ichthyosis, acne, and most recently, wrinkles. How does it work? What does it do and, just as importantly, what does it *not* do?

Thanks to Dr. Voorhees and Dr. Kligman we know that Retin-A makes the top layer of the skin thicker, and it makes its rough exterior smoother and more compact. Retin-A also penetrates into the dermis (the second layer of the skin) where it widens blood vessels and stimulates the formation of new collagen. Frank Chytil, Ph.D., Professor of Biochemistry at Vanderbilt University Medical Center in Nashville, Tennessee, and one of the world's experts on Retin-A biochemistry and metabolism, is the first to admit that we don't know very much about the exact mechanism of action of Retin-A. How does it enter the cells of the skin? Nobody knows for sure. High concentrations seem to have one effect, while lower concentrations have another. Why? And those aren't the only unanswered questions about how it works.

> **Retin-A penetrates into the dermis (the second layer of the skin) where it widens blood vessels and stimulates the formation of new collagen.**

But, as Dr. Chytil's work testifies, despite our lack of knowledge of its exact mechanism of action, there is lots we do know about Retin-A. We have already discovered its effect on over thirty biochemical compounds that are produced by the genes. Some are well known, like insulin and collagen; others are more esoteric, like prolyl-4-hydroxylase and nucleosomal protein. It is clear that Retin-A affects enzymes, receptors, proteins, surface antigens, . . . you name it. That is why the Retin-A picture is so complicated. With the breadth of its impact on important bodily processes, it is difficult—sometimes it seems almost impossible—to ever know or understand all of its ramifications. But research on it marches on.

Retin-A's effectiveness goes well beyond the treatment of ichthyosis, acne, and wrinkles. A multitude of reports have been published about Retin-A's effectiveness on various skin disorders. It has been suggested that it helps over fifty different skin problems. Some of these reports are elaborate clinical evaluations of Retin-A's effectiveness in psoriasis, lichen planus, and warts. Others come from anecdotal and sometimes accidental experiences. For example, a dermatologist in Amarillo, Texas, ob-

> **It has been suggested that Retin-A helps in over fifty different skin problems.**

served that his colleague had used Retin-A with some success on a patient whose skin had been damaged by x-rays. Knowing that he himself had three such damaged areas on his hand and fingers, he decided to try the treatment. Within four weeks of use there was a noticeable improvement in skin texture as well as a decrease in tenderness. Was it the formation of new collagen that achieved the response? We don't know. But the Retin-A worked.

Several interesting projects have proven Retin-A's usefulness in the treatment of pigment disorders. It has been used on melasma, the so-called "mask of pregnancy" (see chapter 4). When Retin-A is used alone or in combination with bleaching creams, it does seem to lighten these areas somewhat. The mechanism by which Retin-A is effective in melasma is very likely similar to or the same as that involved in what Dr. Voorhees found with respect to its ability to lighten age spots.

The list goes on. Precancerous growths, tongue problems, freckles, and even fungus infections like tinea versicolor have been found to be ameliorated. What can't this drug improve?

Retin-A will not remove moles, not deep ones or superficial ones. The reason is that the cells that make up moles are situated in the second layer of the skin or at least very far down in the first layer. Not only are these cells deep, but they are seemingly resistant to Retin-A's many actions. Other growths and tumors will not respond to Retin-A either. Disorders of inflammation, such as lupus, poison ivy rash, or allergies to cosmetics will actually be irritated by Retin-A. Eczema, a very common skin problem in children and adults, will not respond to Retin-A and, in fact, will be irritated by it.

How to Use Retin-A

Retin-A is a prescription drug. If your doctor feels that it is appropriate for you, he or she will then decide on the strength you should start with. But a drug can't work if you don't use it correctly—too much, too little, too often, not often enough. And with Retin-A, rules about usage are *extremely* important, for the amount of the exposure your skin gets to Retin-A is very much a factor with respect to minimizing side effects and maximizing effectiveness. That is why it is available in a number of different strengths and formulations.

The weakest strength is 0.01 percent, followed by 0.025 percent, 0.05 percent, and the strongest strength—0.1 percent. But the percentage can be deceiving. The vehicle, or base (like a cream or a gel) in which the Retin-A is formulated also affects how it's tolerated. Many people find the 0.01 percent *gel* to be harsher than the 0.05 percent *cream*, despite the fact that the percentage concentration of Retin-A is lower in the 0.01 percent gel. The reason for this is that gels are more drying than creams. Because of the above and because people are very sensitive to Retin-A, its use in treatment must be tailored very specifically for the many different skin types and sensitivities that exist. Hence the numerous different combinations of strengths and bases available. Variation in percentage strength and base is also related to what it is being used to treat. Wrinkles dictate one regimen, acne another.

> The physician must tailor the use of Retin-A very specifically to the many different skin types and sensitivities that exist.

But some general principles do exist:

1 ▶ *Wash your face thoroughly.* This removes all of the surface oils and some of the dead cells that may prevent the penetration of Retin-A into the skin. Then wait at least twenty minutes after washing and drying your face before you apply the cream or gel. Although this is the general rule of thumb on how to proceed, individual differences exist. As a result, your dermatologist may suggest certain variations in usage.

Writing in a professional journal, a dermatologist from Warren, Ohio, recently related that a patient of his could not tolerate even the mildest Retin-A preparation and developed dry, flaky, itchy skin even when using it just twice a week. However, when she stopped washing her face before applying Retin-A, she was able to use the cream on a nightly basis. Often, finding the right way to use Retin-A requires close observation and cooperation between doctor and patient, and a careful but experimental attitude.

2 ▶ *Only a pea-sized amount should be used to cover the entire area of the face.* People tend to think that if a little bit is good, then much more is great. Not so with Retin-A. You'll be wasting your medicine and your money and inviting more irritation. Just rub a pea-sized amount in so that it penetrates. The same rules apply whether you are using it for acne, wrinkles, or epidermolytic hyperkeratosis.

Retin-A may be applied anywhere on the face, but you have to use caution when applying it to the facial areas that are the most sensitive, namely around the eyes, the mouth, and the nose. In fact, it might be wise to use a weaker preparation for the eyelids and a stronger one for the face. (Yes, Retin-A can be used on the eyelids, but very cautiously.) Dr. Kligman has stated that no harm is done when small amounts of Retin-A enter the eyes or gets on the lips. But it might sting a bit.

3 ▶ *Apply Retin-A at night.* Night application is the way to go with Retin-A for 99 percent of people for whom it is prescribed. This is because Retin-A can react with the sun to produce increased irritation and, as will be discussed later, potentially even more serious problems. However, Dr. Kligman suggests a somewhat more aggressive approach for certain groups of people. His recommendation is to apply Retin-A twice a day— once in the afternoon and once at night—in dark-skinned individuals and in the elderly. This, because as people age, their skin is less able to become inflamed. (This is part of the reason why you rarely see poison ivy dermatitis in elderly persons.) Therefore, the odds of Retin-A being too harsh in an elderly person are less than those for younger people.

> Apply Retin-A at night because it can react with the sun to produce increased irritation.

But for the rest of the population, for whom only nightly use is recommended, one question that arises is, Does that mean every night? Some people, when they first start using it, can't tolerate nightly use. As a result, some just give up using Retin-A. My approach is to ease them into nightly use. I often have them begin using Retin-A twice a week. If that goes well, I then increase it to three times, then four times, until they work up to every night. Some people, however, can't ever reach the point where they are able to tolerate Retin-A used every night. As long as it does the job, it's fine if you plateau at four or five times a week. However, it takes time before you can make an evaluation. For acne, you should know within a month if the Retin-A treatment is going to work. For wrinkles, it could take six months before any results are seen.

4 ▶ *Don't apply Retin-A when you have any other topical preparations on the facial skin.* Dr. Kligman explains why. Retin-A can be incompatible with other substances, especially fragrances and preservatives. This is easy enough advice to follow. Since the vast majority of people use Retin-A at night, there should be no need to apply makeup at that time. If nighttime moisturizers are used, they can be applied at least thirty to forty-five minutes *after* the application of Retin-A.

Don't apply Retin-A when you have any other topical preparations on the facial skin—it can be incompatible with other substances, especially fragrances and preservatives.

5 ▶ *Wash off the Retin-A first thing in the morning.* This is so important, because you mustn't go out into the sun with Retin-A on your face. And, once you've washed your face you are then also perfectly free to put on any other creams, drugs, or makeup.

But, again, let me emphasize that you not use knowledge of these general principles to avoid what is essential to a successful outcome with Retin-A, and that you and your doctor work together to arrive at just the right dosage for you. Differences between having sensitive or tough skin, between being nineteen or ninety, coming from one part of the country or another—they all affect your treatment regimen.

Writing in the *Journal of the American Medical Association* in December of 1988, Karen Elizabeth Burke, M.D., and Gloria F. Graham, M.D., discussed differences in the way Retin-A is prescribed for use with patients in rural North Carolina from the way its use is prescribed for patients living in urban Manhattan—differences that take into account variations in such factors as their likely diagnoses, the weather, their work and leisure activities, and their appearance expectations.

For the North Carolina farmer with numerous precancerous spots, Drs. Burke and Graham recommended using Retin-A twice a day, despite the redness and peeling that may result. For the New Yorker who wants improvement for wrinkles but will barely tolerate any redness, there is a different regimen. A low-dose Retin-A cream or gel is recommended for use every other night on the entire face, with touchup applications directly on the wrinkles on the off-nights.

Length of Treatment

The length of time that one uses Retin-A depends on what is being treated. Simple acne problems may go away in six months or less. Lifelong congenital disorders, such as ichthyosis, may require lifelong treatments.

Most experts agree that, regarding wrinkles, Retin-A is a forever thing: in order to remove the ravages of the sun and time and then continue to keep them at bay, you must continue to use Retin-A. Dr. Kligman recommends using the standard treatment program for up to one year, after which he begins a maintenance schedule, which involves using Retin-A at bedtime, either on a Monday-Wednesday-Friday schedule or a Saturday-Sunday schedule. Alan Shalita, M.D., chairman of the Dermatology Department at Downstate Medical Center in Brooklyn, New York, disagrees. He feels that most adults prefer daily low-dose maintenance schedules. You and your physician will determine what's right for you.

> In order to remove the ravages of the sun and time—and to keep them at bay—you must continue to use Retin-A.

Side Effects of Retin-A

No drug comes without side effects. Retin-A's most common side effect is that of skin irritation, which takes the form of redness, scaling, and itching. You will recall that in Dr. Voorhees's landmark study, just about every one of the participants (92 percent) experienced irritation from Retin-A, although not all of them experienced it for the full duration of the treatment. It should be remembered, in connection with the side effect rate, that they were using the strongest strength cream—0.1 percent. Even so, based on my experience and that of others, this seems to be an unusually high number of irritant reactions. Recall also that only 8 percent of those in the study withdrew due to the side effects. Thus, the side effects could not have been so very disturbing. Kligman, in his study of four hundred women, used either medium strength, 0.05 percent, cream or full strength, 0.1 percent, cream. He reported that only mild irritation was seen, and it occurred only for the first month in about 25 percent of the participants. Of those, most had fair skin. Although no one has looked at the methods employed or the nature of the participants themselves to come up with an explanation for the rather large difference in the percentage of people who are reported to have experienced side effects—25 percent in the Kligman study and 92 percent in the Voorhees study—some facts are clear. The weakest strengths—0.025 percent and 0.01 percent, yield the lowest likelihood of irritation. Virtually nobody gets irritated from the weaker strengths, whereas some to all experience irritation with the stronger strengths. As discussed above, the variation at the stronger strength is affected by skin type and sensitivity, and age.

One thing to keep in mind when using Retin-A is that it will make you more sensitive to the sun. Therefore, not only should you use sunscreen, you must also be careful about which medications you take. Certain drugs are photosensitizers—they make the skin extra sensitive to the sun. The very commonly used diuretic hydrochlorothiazide is a photosensitizer. A milder photosensitizer is the antibiotic tetracycline. Because it is the most frequently used antibiotic for treating acne, and Retin-A is used for acne, the two of them will often be prescribed for the same person. When this occurs, or when any drug that acts as a photosensitizer is used when you are using Retin-A, extra precautions should be taken against the sun. This is a good example of the general rule to always tell your doctor all the topical and oral drugs you are already using. It helps the physician make the proper diagnosis and select a treatment that won't complicate other medical problems or interact badly with other medicines you are taking.

Retin-A can make you more sensitive to the sun.

Retin-A can, very occasionally, cause a temporary lightening or darkening of the skin. There has been only one report of any scarring following application of Retin-A. It happened to a Canadian woman who used a 0.05 percent gel (which is not available in the United States) on her face four times a day. Yes, you read it right, *four* times a day! By the time things healed two weeks later, superficial scars were present on the face. As Daniel J. Hogan, M.D., of the University of Saskatchewan has pointed out, there is no need for redness or scaling to occur in order to benefit from Retin-A use. It is a matter of finding the minimum therapeutic dosage. And this will vary at different stages of treatment. Keeping this in mind is especially important since gross overuse can lead to more than just discomfort, as the story about the Canadian woman shows.

Is there any danger involved in using Retin-A during pregnancy? It has been found that when it is applied to the skin it penetrates the epidermis and accumulates in the dermis. Very little of this drug gets absorbed into the system. Dr. T. C. Chiang of the Johnson and Johnson Research Center proved this ten years ago. He had volunteers apply Retin-A cream twice a day to their entire body. After a whole month of doing so, the blood levels of Retin-A were measured. Neither Retin-A nor any of its breakdown products could be found. There has never been a case of birth defects associated with it.

So does a pregnant woman have the green light regarding Retin-A? At a special symposium at the Forty-seventh Annual Meeting of the American Academy of Dermatology, on December 6, 1988, almost one year after the Voorhees results had been announced, Dr. Voorhees's group, while agreeing with the above points, nevertheless recommended *not* to prescribe Retin-A to pregnant women. Dr. Kligman, writing just a few months earlier in the *Journal of the American Medical Association*, addressed the same issue in an article entitled "Is Topical Tretinoin Teratogenic [capable of causing malformations in a fetus]?". He concluded that in view of the laboratory and clinical evidence available, Retin-A was safe to use during pregnancy.

In an important article published in the *Journal of the American Academy of Dermatology* on the use of oral and topical agents for acne during pregnancy, Peter Pochi, M.D., and Karen Rothman, M.D., from the Department of Dermatology at Boston University stated that, should a woman become pregnant while using Retin-A, the ultimate decision to continue its use should be made by the woman and her obstetrician. They noted that there has never been a report of an abnormal offspring from the use of this drug in pregnancy.

Where does that leave us? Despite the varying conclusions reported above, the clinical evidence suggests that Retin-A is safe for use in pregnancy. This was supported by a 1993 article in the well-respected British medical journal *Lancet*: the study showed that using Retin-A in the first three months of pregnancy had no effect on the baby and no increase in birth defects. The decision to continue or start using Retin-A in pregnancy depends on how conservative or liberal the patient and the doctor are with regard to drug use. Part of the decision will obviously have to do with how serious is the problem for which the Retin-A is being considered as a treatment.

There appears to be some new evidence that long-term use of Retin-A might lead to a previously unreported side effect. Some investigators have pointed to growing suspicions that too much Retin-A can create a mat of dilated blood vessels on the face. We learned earlier from the work of Dr. Voorhees and others that

Retin-A can give the skin a rosy glow. It apparently accomplishes this by widening the blood vessels. Other researchers, such as Dr. Kligman, feel that new blood vessels are formed. Reports suggest that this impact on the blood vessels is what's responsible for giving the face a rosy color, which can be quite desirable. But this very same mechanism can also be responsible for causing the development of frankly visible veins. This side effect is hardly desirable. Fortunately, it is quite uncommon. What all this suggests, however, is that further investigation is still needed concerning strength used, frequency of dosage, and duration of treatment with respect to effectiveness and specific side effects of Retin-A.

There is another concern. Retin-A has been shown to produce skin cancer in *animals*. In different studies by independent investigators, Retin-A in combination with ultraviolet light led to the formation of skin cancer in hairless mice. The exact mechanism by which Retin-A induces these skin cancers in animals is still unknown. Some experts feel that the DNA of the cells is affected. Others feel that it is by altering epidermal growth that it causes skin cancer. Another possible mechanism suggested is related to something that Dr. Voorhees had demonstrated in his early study— that Retin-A made the epidermis thicker. Perhaps by some means or another, when Retin-A is combined with ultraviolet light it might cause the epidermis to grow in an uncontrolled manner into skin cancer.

But how does that tally with what was stated earlier—that Retin-A has a *beneficial* effect on precancerous skin lesions? For, Retin-A has been shown to cause tumor regression in mice and has a beneficial effect on precancerous actinic keratoses. How do we explain this apparent paradox? The difference may depend on the concentration of Retin-A, the amount of ultraviolet exposure, or other unknown factors. According to John Epstein, M.D., of the Department of Dermatology at the University of California, San Francisco, although both negative and positive effects of Retin-A on skin tumors have been demonstrated in animals, there has never been a case of skin cancer reported in humans.

All of these concerns were on the minds of top researchers who gathered for an international symposium on Retin-A and related compounds. It was April of 1986 in New York City, a little less than two years before the Voorhees results were announced. Presentations were given and discussions ensued. One attendee asked the panel of experts, "The thing that concerns me is that John Epstein tells us that under certain conditions, tretinoin (the chemical name for Retin-A) can produce skin cancer, and under other conditions it won't. Are we going to produce skin cancers in the elderly if we keep rubbing this stuff on?"

Dr. Lorraine Kligman (Dr. Albert Kligman's wife and collaborator) was the first to respond. She made it clear that the hairless mouse model was a very relevant animal for testing the capability of a substance to produce *or* protect against skin cancers. However, to the question at hand she answered that no teenager using Retin-A had ever developed a tumor. Dr. Epstein agreed with Dr. Kligman that we had no evidence that retinoic acid was carcinogenic in humans. But he added, "Although I don't know that it will not be a tumor promoter in older people, I suggest it probably won't."

We thus do not have a definitive answer, and because of that, not everyone is breathing more easily. David Bickers, M.D., chairman of the Department of Dermatology at Case Western Reserve University in Cleveland, Ohio, appeared on the television program "60 Minutes," February 4, 1990, the same program we mentioned earlier. He expressed concerns about long-term safety. Dr. Bickers said that treating acne in teenagers for a *few* months to years is different than treating wrinkles in adults for *many* years. The results from one situation may not apply to the other.

The history of medicine provides us with good reasons to worry about long-term side effects of new therapies. One of the many such stories is the following. About sixty years ago, doctors found a new treatment for acne, rashes, and fungus. Sometimes just a few treatments were necessary, sometimes quite a few. But eventually the treatments worked. The populace had never seen such a wonderful treatment. It was called x-ray therapy. The rest, as they say, is history. And not very happy history. For it wasn't until twenty to thirty years later that doctors discovered that the doses used for treating such skin conditions could cause cancer. By then, for many, it was too late.

Hence, we are left with a basic question—should people worry that they will be carrying around a face full of skin cancers just because they used Retin-A for wrinkles? In view of all the preceding evidence, based upon twenty years of patient use, it seems safe to say that Retin-A does not promote the formation of skin cancer. I would tend to agree with the majority of experts who vouch for the long-term safety of Retin-A. But it is clear that carefully designed studies are really needed to finally put the issue to rest. For, although we have been prescribing Retin-A for twenty years there have been no studies of people who themselves have used Retin-A for various long-term periods—studies which would be able to establish whether or not the likelihood of any side effects, like cancer, exists.

The Alpha-Hydroxy-Acids (AHAs)

Retin-A is not the only new topical method of treating wrinkles, age spots, and other common cosmetic problems. The alpha-hydroxy-acids (AHAs) are now attracting a great deal of attention. Although their pharmacological roots are ancient, the AHAs are the new wonder drug of the 1990s. Because they showed success with some of the same skin problems treated successfully with Retin-A, comparisons have been inevitable.

A very interesting comparison between the two has to do with the striking similarities in how long it took each of them to become acknowledged as an antiwrinkle agent. Retin-A, as you recall, was first introduced in the early 1960s for the treatment of acne but didn't get recognized as a savior for wrinkled faces until *twenty-five* years later. Similarly, the AHAs were being used for dry skin for a period of almost *twenty* years before their effects on wrinkled skin became widely known.

This kind of delay is not unfamiliar in medicine. A drug can be in use for a while for *one* purpose, and, later, its beneficial effects for *another* ailment will emerge. Research must then be conducted on its safety and effectiveness for this new use. The rigorous, scientific testing that is required and the publication of the results of these studies can take years. Then the FDA has to approve that same drug for its safety and effectiveness in treating the new problem. This slow, conservative, painstaking process is one that increases the likelihood that the results will be sound and reliable. Sometimes, when treatments or drugs are approved more quickly—as with some drugs for AIDS—it stirs controversy. The question arises: Was enough care given to determine their safety and/or effectiveness? For, early in medical school we are taught: "Above all else, do no harm"—and the field of medicine holds tenaciously to that dictum. If waiting a few more years gets the kinks out of a drug, then it is usually worth it.

Some Background

Recognition of the effectiveness of the AHAs is due to the work of Eugene Van Scott, M.D., of Abington, Pennsylvania, and formerly affiliated with the Department of Dermatology at Temple University in Philadelphia as well as the National Institutes of Health. He has been studying AHAs since the early 1970s and is to the AHAs what his cross-town colleague, Dr. Kligman, at the University of Pennsylvania, is to Retin-A.

> The AHAs are found in many natural plant sources, including sugar cane, lemons, and old wine.

The AHAs have one advantage over Retin-A in the treatment of wrinkles and age spots. They are natural. They can be found in the human body and in many other plant sources, such as sugar cane and lemons. In our day and age of artificial everything, a naturally occurring treatment is quite welcome.

The AHAs are a group of several different acids that bear certain chemical similarities. Some of these acids are quite familiar to all of us. Citric acid is found in citrus fruits, such as oranges and lemons. Another one that is common is lactic acid. Less well known is malic acid, found in apples. Two more AHAs are tartaric acid and glycolic acid. Old wine is rich in tartaric acid, and it has been claimed that the women of the European nobility used old wine on their faces to smooth out their skin.

Before the introduction of cortisone creams in the 1950s, natural remedies were the mainstay of topical dermatologic treatment. Many of you will remember creams, lotions, and ointments containing mercury, such as Mercurochrome. Iodine, a common natural ingredient in seafood, continues to be a popular topical skin disinfectant to this day. Compounds with sulfur were also demonstrated to have therapeutic value.

With the 1950s came the synthetic age. In addition to cortisone creams, newer antibiotics, both oral and topical, were introduced. The natural skin remedies were becoming a threatened species. But "natural" decided to make a comeback. The use of natural remedies is well accepted in modern day dermatology. The 1970s saw the emergence of interest in aloe vera. Aloe is a plant species that is widely grown. The ancient Chinese used extracts of the aloe plant over two thousand years ago to treat stomach disorders. The South American and Central American Indians still use aloe gel in the treatment of skin diseases (see chapter 5 for more on aloe vera). Thus, the use of the natural AHAs as a treatment has historical precedent.

In 1974 Dr. Van Scott and Ruey J. Yu, Ph.D., published an important article in a top dermatology journal, the *Archives of Dermatology*. Entitled "Control of Keratinization with Alpha-Hydroxy-Acids and Related Compounds," this article demonstrated how ichthyosis (the "alligator skin" disorder) could be remarkably cleared by applying several different fruit acids to the skin in an ointment form. In the ensuing years, further studies done by Drs. Van Scott and Yu were able to show how the AHAs were helpful in the treatment of disorders whose primary symptom is dry skin. Psoriasis, eczema, and dry skin not associated with any particular condition or disease were all shown to be ameliorated by the AHAs.

The AHAs help with disorders whose primary symptom is dry skin, like psoriasis and eczema.

However, as Dr. Van Scott's material appeared in one periodical after another, some people wondered why no one else was engaging in research on the AHAs. Then, in early 1990, researchers from a major California medical center announced some impressive results with glycolic acid, the foremost AHA. One hundred and fifty patients were treated for wrinkles, age spots, and other untoward effects of sun and aging. Those that were treated with glycolic acid showed marked improvement. Howard Murad, M.D., the senior member of the research team, reported that a high concentration of glycolic acid was applied to the face for a few minutes, and then it was washed off. The application caused some burning or stinging. Following this treatment, over the next few days, the dry skin dissolved and the skin assumed a rosy color. The patients maintained this improvement by then using a lower concentration of glycolic acid at home. But Dr. Murad felt that it might be best if the stronger concentration of glycolic acid were to be reapplied in the dermatologist's office from every few weeks in some cases up to every few months in others.

As if wrinkles and age spots weren't enough to claim benefits for, Dr. Murad praised the effect that glycolic acid had on acne as well. Pores became unplugged, whiteheads and blackheads were expressed, or "spurt out," and a better complexion resulted. Dr. Murad also found that a medium strength concentration was very useful for thickened skin on the palms and soles.

Dr. Van Scott had conducted his own study on twenty-seven women who were treated with a slightly different technique for applying AHAs—minipeels (see below) and maintenance therapy for wrinkles. After three months, twenty-one were improved, nine experienced mild-to-moderate improvement, while twelve experienced substantial improvement.

The AHAs: Their Mode of Action

When Drs. Van Scott and Yu published their 1974 study (referred to earlier), they studied a dozen different AHAs to see what AHAs do to the skin. They found that the AHAs' most remarkable effect is on the outermost part of the skin, the stratum corneum, which is the compact layer of keratin cells that lies above the epidermis (described in chapter 2). In conditions such as psoriasis, ichthyosis (alligator skin), or just plain dry skin, the stratum corneum is vastly thickened. This can be due to one of two things—either the overproduction of the keratin cells or the decreased ability to shed the cells once they are formed.

> The AHAs' most remarkable effect is on the outermost part of the skin—the stratum corneum.

It has been noted that certain disorders of the stratum corneum, often referred to as hyperkeratosis, tend to improve in the warm summer months, when the air is more humid. Conversely, in those areas of the country where the winter months are cold and there is lower humidity and stronger winds, the skin becomes drier. With less humidity in the air, less moisture is available to the stratum corneum.

That's why moisturizers—which deliver water to the stratum corneum—are used to treat disorders of hyperkeratosis. Yet, they do not provide the total answer. The symptoms generally still persist, even if in somewhat diminished a form. As an example of the limited benefits of moisturizing on this condition, it has been demonstrated that fetuses that have inherited ichthyosis already have their "alligator" skin in their mothers' wombs, despite the fact that their skin is surrounded by liquid (amniotic fluid) all of the time. So, if 100 percent humidity can't moisturize dry skin, what can?

The AHAs provide an answer. They exert their effect on the newly forming keratin cells at the bottom of the stratum corneum. This causes the bulk of the stratum corneum to lift off and separate from the underlying skin. As a result the stratum corneum becomes much thinner. This gives the skin a much smoother look and feel.

Not only that, but a thin stratum corneum bends more easily than a thick one, so that cracking and fissuring are minimized as well.

You might recall that Dr. Voorhees's study of Retin-A showed that it, too, reduces the thickness of the stratum corneum. But the effects of Retin-A on the horny layer are not nearly as remarkable as the effects of the AHAs. That is because they work by different mechanisms. Although the precise manner in which these agents act has not been worked out to 100 percent certainty, it appears that the AHAs weaken the strength of the horny layer by stopping the synthesis of the material that functions like glue to hold the cells together. In other words, the AHAs shut down the "glue manufacturing plant." Retin-A, on the other hand, works by breaking down the glue that is already there. Apparently decreasing the manufacture of that glue is ultimately a more effective way to decrease the scaliness of the skin.

In their 1974 study, Drs. Van Scott and Yu demonstrated another interesting effect of the AHAs on the epidermis. They found that the epidermis of patients with ichthyosis who were treated with AHAs actually decreased in thickness, just as the stratum corneum did. This is in marked contrast to Retin-A which, as Dr. Voorhees showed, significantly increases the thickness of the epidermis. Why the difference? Part of the answer may lie in the AHAs' effect on the breakdown of sugar in the skin. Certain sugars and their enzymes play a major role in keeping the cells of the skin cemented (glued) together. Disrupting the cement can cause parts of the skin to become weaker, which could then lead to thinning.

One thing that we do know is that when the AHAs are applied in higher concentrations to the skin, they cause epidermolysis. As the name suggests, this is the lysis (splitting) of the epidermis. The subsequent sloughing of the skin gives the remaining skin a smoother look. It is by this same mechanism that the AHAs get rid of age spots and precancerous growths. There are limits as to how thin or thick the epidermis gets in response to these medications. The AHAs do not thin out the epidermis completely, nor does constant use of Retin-A make the skin as thick as an elephant's. Each reaches a plateau and stays there.

As with Retin-A, the AHAs' least understood effects are their impact on the dermis. However, Dr. Van Scott suspects that it is in this layer of skin where the AHAs exert their antiwrinkle effects. Preliminary evidence indicates that the AHAs may turn on the synthesis (the production) of dermal glycosaminoglycans. That's a big word, so let me explain.

In a nutshell, the dermis itself is composed of three main parts: (1) collagen, (2) elastic fibers, and (3) ground substances. Glycosaminoglycans are the major components of ground substances. By beefing up the ground substance, the dermis becomes thicker, thereby eradicating wrinkles. Not only that, but ascorbic acid—one of the AHAs—has been demonstrated to promote collagen synthesis in human skin. Dr. Van Scott feels that by increasing the amounts of two of the three components of human dermis—the ground substances and the collagen—the AHAs can really counter the mechanics of wrinkling.

> By increasing the amounts of the ground substances and the collagen in the dermis, the AHAs can really counter the mechanics of wrinkling.

Keep in mind that both Dr. Voorhees and Dr. Kligman showed that Retin-A also increased the amount of collagen in the dermis. However, neither has been able to determine the exact mechanism by which this happens with Retin-A.

One interesting difference between the AHAs and Retin-A is that the human body can produce AHAs on its own. It can't produce Retin-A since this compound is derived from vitamin A, which is not produced by the body. (Vitamin A occurs naturally outside the human body in many plants, some of which serve as food sources for this nutrient.)

But although the body produces AHAs, these obviously don't do the job we'd like them to in regard to preventing wrinkles. Probably one of the main reasons for this, maybe *the* reason, is revealed, again, by the work done by Dr. Van Scott. His research indicates that the body also produces acids that are *antagonistic* to the AHAs' effects, namely, the alpha-acetoxy-acids, or the AAAs. Studies have shown that the AAAs work in manner that is opposite to the AHAs—they make both the stratum corneum and epidermis thicker while, as discussed above, the AHAs make these two skin layers thinner. Instead of smoothing out the skin, the AAAs cause it to become rougher and permit more blackheads and whiteheads to form. The natural, inborn antagonism, or opposition, between these two acids probably serves to keep a balance between the stratum corneum and the epidermis.

In sum, the AHAs and Retin-A do not work precisely in the same way on the skin. Differences exist on every layer, even though both compounds have been proven effective for a variety of similar skin disorders.

The AHAs: Virtues and Limits

Several years ago, a prescription product was introduced that contained 12 percent lactic acid (one of the AHAs) for the treatment of dry skin disorders. Innovative dermatologists, however, soon found that it also helped with skin problems such as keratosis pilaris—a condition where hundreds of little spiny bumps form on the upper arms and sometimes on the cheeks and thighs. By applying the lactic acid lotion, the keratin plugs are loosened and the skin that was once like cobblestone becomes smooth again. Over-the-counter lactic acid lotions and creams can also be helpful.

The newer age of AHA treatment revolves around the application of high concentration AHAs to specific problem areas on the skin. The class of skin problems called the keratoses is a good example. Actinic keratosis involves the precancerous spots we discussed earlier (see chapters 3 and 8). Another form of keratosis, seborrheic keratosis (chapter 3), produces the most common benign skin growth in America. These are brown, stubbly bumps that are usually concentrated on the trunk of people forty-five years of age and older. Dr. Kligman and Dr. Van Scott concur that most age spots on the face are really mild forms of seborrheic keratoses, making them quite suitable to treatment with high concentration AHAs.

The procedure for using an AHA for removal of a keratosis is often referred to as a "spot peel." A high concentration AHA is applied to the affected spot only, not the area around it. Concentrations of 70 percent to 100 percent are used—doses that are available to physicians only. This is carefully applied to each keratosis, skillfully avoiding spillage onto the normal surrounding skin. After three to four minutes, the keratosis is usually saturated. If not, a second application may be necessary. The result of this process is that a lesion that was once firm and crusty is now soft and rubbery. It can then easily be removed by curettage—a gentle scraping of the skin with a blunt instrument. Although a burning sensation can occur, it is usually mild. The skin is then cleansed with water or sodium bicarbonate solution to eliminate any acid that might remain on the skin. With this spot peel method, scores of keratoses can be removed in one sitting.

Even at significantly lower concentrations, home use for this purpose has come into disfavor. Dr. Van Scott gave several patients the opportunity to use concentrations of 25 to 40 percent to treat their keratoses at home. The solutions were dispensed only to those who had demonstrated that they could follow instructions carefully and understood the dangers of noncompliance. The concentrated AHAs were to be applied twice a day by the patient or a family member. They were instructed to use the solution for one to three days. Some patients did quite well, and the keratosis gradually separated or withered away. Other patients, despite their caution, were not as fortunate. They quickly came back into the doctor's office with redness and peeling of the normal skin surrounding the keratosis. Dr. Van Scott came to an important conclusion that has since been supported by others. The use of highly concentrated AHAs should only be done by a doctor.

> The use of highly concentrated AHAs should only be done by a doctor.

The AHAs work very well with acne. When the acne is on the chest or back, solutions of 40 to 70 percent are used. The solution is spread with a cotton ball uniformly over the affected area. Within three to five minutes, the whiteheads, blackheads, pustules, and bumps begin to blanch. Some pimples may even pop open as a result of the disintegration of the overlying stratum corneum. The area is then rinsed with water or bicarbonate, just as with the treatment of a keratosis. The doctor must employ caution so as not to leave the solution on for too long. To do so can leave the area looking red for several days. When done correctly, the procedure can be repeated anywhere from every week to every month.

For acne on the face, a similar approach is used. Redness may last an hour or two, followed by mild peeling, which can persist for up to forty-eight hours. Home use of a 5 or 10 percent AHA lotion can reinforce the use of the stronger solution used by the physician for a minipeel.

The effect of the AHAs on wrinkles is their crowning glory. For the treatment of wrinkles, a 70 percent glycolic acid solution is applied every few weeks. High-strength glycolic acid has been found to be the most effective AHA for this purpose. At each application, the face is cleaned with an antibacterial soap and then the glycolic acid is applied with cotton tipped applicators. It is left on a little bit longer than in the acne treatments—about four to ten minutes. The skin is then washed off with water or bicarbonate. As the patient's skin becomes acclimated to the treatments, the glycolic acid can be left on for longer periods of time in order to enhance results. In between treatments, a 10 percent glycolic acid gel is used twice a day. As when they are used for acne, when glycolic acid peels are used for wrinkles they may leave the face red for a few days. And, again, as in the case of acne treatment, minipeel patients should use a 10 percent glycolic acid gel for maintenance. Lactic acid preparations may also be helpful.

Suffice it to say that the glycolic acid minipeels for wrinkles do have certain advantages and drawbacks relative to the other types of acid peels. (See also the section below on Chemical Peels.)

How to Use the AHAs

As with Retin-A, different strengths of the AHAs are available. A very important difference between Retin-A and the AHAs is that Retin-A is available by prescription only. The AHAs, on the other hand, are either over-the-counter or prescription preparations, depending on how concentrated they are. A commonly used AHA for home application is glycolic acid. It usually comes in 8 to 10 percent strengths, which are available without a prescription. Over-the-counter lactic acid products are available in strengths from 2.5 to 5 percent. A 12 percent strength of lactic acid is available for home use, but it is available by prescription only.

The AHAs come in creams, gels, or lotions. Some of glycolic acid preparations are combined with hydroquinone, a bleaching agent, which adds to the effectiveness of the AHA in the treatment of age spots and the mask of pregnancy.

Just as there were rules for the usage of Retin-A, so are there for the AHAs. Some are the same, some are different:

1 ▶ *Wash the face thoroughly*: Washing removes surface oils that may hinder AHA penetration. Also, a stratum corneum that has been hydrated (moisturized by washing the skin) allows for better penetration of the AHAs. The greater the penetration, the greater the effect.

2 ▶ *Use only as much as you need*: Creams, gels, and lotions vary in consistency. Therefore, you will find yourself using different amounts of each. Using six layers is, however, no more effective than using just one. Use enough to cover the skin and then rub it in. There is usually less sensitivity around the eyes to the AHAs than to Retin-A. Not that the AHA compounds should be used without care around the eyes, for they will sting.

3 ▶ *Use twice or three times a day*: This is quite different from Retin-A therapy. The reason for the difference is that the AHAs have virtually no interaction with the sun. Therefore, they can be used in the daytime as well as at night. For maintenance treatment of acne or wrinkles, glycolic acid in a 10 percent concentration is used twice a day. For more extensive disorders, such as ichthyosis, lactic acid in a 12 percent concentration may be used three or four times a day. Most people can begin using the AHAs twice a day right from the start. Unlike Retin-A, which usually requires a breaking-in period, the AHAs seem to be well tolerated. Retin-A is simply a harsher medication and needs to be introduced more gradually.

> The AHAs can be used in the daytime as well as at night because, unlike Retin-A, they have virtually no interaction with the sun.

Because the use of AHAs under medical supervision is still new, no long-term studies are available. A twice- or three-times-a-day regimen would seem to suffice for most common disorders.

It appears that fair-skinned people are able to use the AHAs as readily as those with darker complexions. Dr. Van Scott advocates using the AHAs on a daily basis for maintenance. Although twice a day is the norm, individual adjustments are in order, depending upon the severity of the condition being treated and the person's own tolerance.

Side Effects of the AHAs

The major determinant of whether you will experience side effects from the AHAs is the strength of the particular product being used. The over-the-counter glycolic acids, which come in 8 to 10 percent strengths, are strong enough to provide good results but too weak to give significant side effects. On the other hand, prescription strength lactic acid (12 percent ammonium lactate) lotion carries with it a bit more irritation. According to the *Physicians' Desk Reference*, the most frequent adverse reactions to it in people with dry skin are as follows (where the percentage indicates percent of the total people studied): transient stinging—3 percent; burning—3 percent; redness—3 percent; peeling—1 percent. From my experience I would think that those percentages should actually be a bit higher, especially in people with cracked or fissured skin.

The 70 percent glycolic acid solutions applied by doctors for minipeels are in an entirely different category. Because they are so strong, they virtually always cause stinging, redness, and peeling. The redness and peeling may last days to weeks. To date, however, I have not heard of anyone developing scarring from this, but I would not be at all surprised to hear of such an unfortunate side effect, especially as this technique gets more widespread use. But, overall, the AHAs tend to be quite safe. This, because as per Dr. Van Scott, they are very physiologic. That is, they are a substance that the human body itself produces. For the most part, studies seem to corroborate his opinion concerning safety. That is not to say that allergic reactions to the AHAs are not possible. Adverse reactions to natural substances are well known, with poison ivy dermatitis and aloe vera allergies being two common examples.

> There have never been any reported cases of scarring with the AHAs: if irritation and redness occur, these reactions are not permanent.

Sun sensitivity, such a prevalent problem with Retin-A, has never been reported with the AHAs. Nor has the prolonged use of glycolic acid (in contrast to Retin-A) resulted in blood vessels showing through the skin, according to Dr. Van Scott. And, as mentioned earlier, there have never been any reported cases of scarring with the AHAs—that is, irritation reactions and redness are not permanent.

Little is known regarding the use of the AHAs in pregnant women. Animal reproduction studies have never been conducted with the 12 percent lactic acid lotion form. The *Physicians' Desk Reference* states that it is not known whether it can cause fetal harm when administered to pregnant women or if reproduction capacity is affected. It concludes that it should be prescribed for pregnant women only if clearly needed. Where does that leave us in regard to weaker strength AHAs, such as the 8 percent or 10 percent lactic or glycolic acids? Dr. Van Scott feels that lower strength AHAs are probably safe during pregnancy.

The main question that remains in terms of adverse reactions concerns the impact of the AHAs on skin cancer formation. Unlike Retin-A, elaborate animal studies have never been carried out to determine whether or not a risk exists. Dr. Van Scott highly doubts whether low concentration AHAs would ever cause skin cancer. He acknowledges, however, that any irritating substance, if used for a long enough time, may act as a promoter of skin cancer. But, he adds, the lower strength AHAs do not irritate and thus would not be considered cancer causing.

In summary, several things can be said. The AHAs have not been as intensely studied as Retin-A. The side-effect profile appears to be safer, but questions regarding pregnancy and long-term adverse effects, like cancer formation, still remain.

Which Is Better, Retin-A or the AHAs?

The above discussion may have you in a quandary. Both preparations sound good. Both work for wrinkles as well as for age spots and keratoses. Both work within a few months. But which one is really better? They both have some downsides. How do you choose? "Higher concentrations of Retin-A seem to be more effective for wrinkles," concedes Dr. Murad. "But," he adds, "these cause more irritations, increase sensitivity to sunlight and may, therefore, promote even greater telangiectasias (dilated blood vessels)."

Dr. Kligman defends Retin-A as being the top of the line. He has also wondered out loud whether the AHAs are overrated. Retin-A has helped millions. "Nothing," says Dr. Kligman, "can beat it." However, Dr. Van Scott thinks otherwise. He feels that the AHAs offer safety and effectiveness that are unparalleled. "Their time has come," he contends.

I asked both Dr. Kligman and Dr. Van Scott what they each thought of using Retin-A and the AHAs together—say, an AHA in the morning and Retin-A at night. Dr. Kligman says that using Retin-A together with the AHAs would lead to an increase in irritation of the skin.

"Increased irritation from Retin-A?" I asked.

"From both," answered Dr. Kligman.

Would the increase in irritation be worth it if you could get better antiwrinkle effects? No, says Dr. Van Scott. He has used Retin-A together with the AHAs and has found no appreciable benefit with the combination therapy.

I also have had a number of patients use both Retin-A and glycolic acid at the same time. Although I would agree with Dr. Van Scott that for some people there may be no great value, there are others who really benefit from the combination therapy. The AHAs in the morning and Retin-A at night seems to work quite well for certain people.

Some Final Observations

There are several things that I have learned about Retin-A and the AHAs from my clinical experience that are nowhere to be found in the textbooks. Occasionally I will have someone tell me that Retin-A "stopped working." There are several possible explanations for this. Certain cosmetics, sunscreens, or even perfumes may interfere with Retin-A's effect. If you have switched to one of them while using Retin-A that new product may interfere. Also, the Retin-A may be past its expiration date. Then, sometimes, people forget to wash their faces before applying Retin-A. In other cases, as with other treatments—both oral and topical—it just stops being effective for no apparent reason. My first response is to either increase the strength of Retin-A or switch to the AHAs. I have heard the same complaint, but less frequently, from people using the AHA glycolic acid. Switching to Retin-A is in order for these people.

There are also reactions to these medications for which we currently have no explanation. I have had several people complain to me that 10 percent glycolic acid lotion aggravates or causes acne, most frequently on the lower cheeks. Careful questioning must be pursued to determine if makeup, perfume, and other factors that can interact with this treatment may be the problem. But more often than not it seems to be just an idiosyncratic reaction to the glycolic acid, with no easy or apparent explanation. Interestingly, if you look up the list of adverse reactions to another one of the AHAs, ammonium lactate 12 percent lotion, acne is not one of them. Once more, clinical experience with a drug proves to be one of the best sources of information about it.

There are some products called Retin-A "enhancers" and Retin-A "strengtheners." These claim to increase penetration while decreasing its side effects, and dermatologists and their patients have been bombarded with advertisements for them. But there are several things to keep in mind when evaluating these products: (1) Ortho Pharmaceuticals, the manufacturer of Retin-A, does not endorse using any of these products together with Retin-A; (2) so far these products have not been evaluated scientifically by top, independent investigators; (3) it is not known whether they penetrate past the stratum corneum or epidermis, what their dermal effects are, or whether they themselves have side effects; and (4) remember the comments of Dr. Kligman and others, who maintain that Retin-A is an unstable compound that may be incompatible with other substances.

People who use glycolic acid exclusively, on an everyday basis, for the control of wrinkles should, as Dr. Murad recommends, get minipeels every few months to maintain their skin tone.

I don't know how many patients of mine have gone to Tijuana, Mexico (where Retin-A is sold without a prescription), and have brought back a product that is less expensive but causes them any number of complications. You simply can't expect that the Retin-A you buy in Mexico will be the same as the product sold in the United States. Keep in mind that this country has very strict quality control standards, which serve to protect you. Don't take chances when it comes to your health or appearance.

> The nonprescription Retin-A sold outside the United States may not meet the high quality control standards we have in this country.

Questions of quality and effectiveness come up with respect to generics also. An important fact to remember is that as of April 1990, Ortho Pharmaceutical's patent on Retin-A expired. Therefore, generic copies of Retin-A will soon become available.

Richard B. Stoughton of the Department of Dermatology at the University of California at San Diego is considered by many to be the foremost authority in the country on evaluating the potency of topical creams and ointments. In October 1987, when the generic drug market was doing a booming business, Dr. Stoughton published an eye-opening article in the *Archives of Dermatology*. He compared the strengths of topical brand-name steroid products and their generic "equivalents." What he found was not so equivalent. In fact, large discrepancies were noted between them. He concluded that doctors should be aware that significant differences in therapeutic effectiveness do occur between some generic and brand-name creams and ointments.

The FDA is well aware of Dr. Stoughton's study and the fact that Retin-A is not just any cream. They have established new rules that will require generic manufacturers to prove with double-blind studies like those of Dr. Voorhees that their product works as well as Retin-A. Only then will they be allowed to market a generic Retin-A. Until all of the kinks are worked out of the generics and until truly independent investigators like Dr. Stoughton can evaluate them, I would recommend that you stick with the real Retin-A.

Watch out for products whose names sound like Retin-A, but aren't. For example, Retinol-A, Rettin-A, and so on. There is only one Retin-A. And it is not available by mail order or "special deals." It is available by prescription only.

Wonder Creams That Never Made It

Aside from Retin-A and the AHAs, many have tried but few have succeeded in producing a cream to reduce wrinkles, age spots, and skin cancer. There is hardly a month that goes by where you don't pick up a paper at the supermarket extolling the virtues of the latest skin remedy. Some are more memorable than others.

Several years ago, a new cream hit the market. The cream contained glycosphingolipid, one of the key ingredients in the nuclei of cells. The claim was simple—use the cream, strengthen your skin, erase those wrinkles forever. Sure, it was expensive, but for what it offered, many felt it was worth it. What's more, it was endorsed by Dr. Christiaan Barnard, the South African surgeon who performed the world's first heart transplant. At the time, he was perhaps the most famous doctor in the entire world. An endorsement from him was sure to get people's attention. Press coverage was enormous. The manufacturers and distributors thought they had a potential gold mine.

Coincidentally, one of my patients owned a renowned testing center for cosmetics. He held a doctoral degree in biochemistry and was known in the industry as an expert on creams, moisturizers, and other similar products. One of the largest and most prestigious companies in the world came to him with the following problem. They were in the mad scramble to get marketing rights for that cream, but before they invested their millions, they wanted to have the cream tested extensively. My patient was happy to oblige them. Hastily, but carefully, he prepared the tests. But when they were completed they all pointed to one conclusion—the cream wasn't what it claimed to be. The company profusely thanked him and withdrew their bid for the marketing rights.

But another company was less cautious and brought the cream out as Glycel. In the ensuing months, heavy media advertising coverage touted Glycel for its miraculous ability to restore youth. Sales soared. Yet, despite the initial excitement, Glycel died a slow death. The scientific community challenged the validity of the cream's claims, and other manufacturers mounted a counter-attack on the truthfulness of Glycel's advertising. The final blow was dealt by the consumers themselves. People simply stopped using Glycel because it turned out to be nothing more than an expensive moisturizer. Eventually it was withdrawn from the market.

Collagen creams have maintained some popularity over the past fifteen years as so-called anti-aging products. Manufacturers claim that rubbing the collagen into your skin replaces the collagen that age and the sun have slowly degraded. Sounds good, except for one thing. It doesn't make any sense scientifically. Most of the collagen extracts have a molecular weight of anywhere from fifteen thousand to fifty thousand daltons. Only substances with a molecular weight of five thousand or less can penetrate the stratum corneum. The collagen in these creams just sits on top of your skin once you apply it. As one expert commented, it's like trying to push a basketball through a hole designed for a Ping-Pong ball.

Certain products have come out that contain an ingredient known as procollagen. Procollagen is chemically similar to collagen. It has the same drawback regarding molecular weight. Unlike Glycel, however, collagen and procollagen creams are not a *total* loss. They do have some beneficial effects on the skin. Collagen creams tend to fill in irregularities on the skin's surface. A protein film forms as they dry, which gives the skin a smooth texture. As the protein film shrinks, it stretches out some of the fine wrinkles and surface irregularities.

The effects of collagen and procollagen creams, however, are short-lived and they must be reapplied constantly to maintain the smoothness. They do not penetrate into the deeper layers of the skin. Actually, the only truly successful collagen treatment for wrinkles is not a cream at all but is *injectable* collagen. Introduced in the early 1970s, injectable collagen has been used on over three hundred thousand people for the treatment of wrinkles and scars. But even injectable collagen must be redone once or twice a year in order to maintain its effect (see below).

One fountain-of-youth cream emerged quite accidentally as a result of noticing the effects on the skin of a chemotherapeutic agent used against cancer—5-fluoro-uracil (5-FU). Very sick cancer patients who were receiving it complained about developing a bothersome rash, which is a common side effect with many anti-cancer (antineoplastic) drugs. But this rash was something special. The rashes occurred on only certain parts of the skin—those portions that had been damaged by the sun. Only the actinic keratoses, those precancerous sun spots discussed earlier, were turning red. The rest of the skin was unaffected. In searching for a reason for this odd occurrence, the physicians concluded that the rash was the result of the sun-damaged cells of the skin absorbing the 5-FU and then being destroyed by it. If 5-FU could wipe out these precancerous lesions on the skin when it was taken orally, researchers wondered if it could do the same when applied topically.

Clinical trials provided them with their answer. It was yes. Their hunch had been correct. And thus, quite accidentally, as often happens in science, a new treatment was born. The effectiveness of 5-FU in treating precancerous growths got people thinking—if an acne medication, such as Retin-A, could turn out to also work for wrinkles, age spots, and precancerous growths, maybe 5-FU, an inhibitor of precancerous growth, could work for acne, wrinkles, and age spots. In fact, as early as 1981, an article by Howard Milstein, M.D., a dermatologist from San Diego, California, was published in the *Journal of the American Academy of Dermatology* attesting to the usefulness of 5-FU as an aid in the management of acne and melasma, the so-called mask of pregnancy. But despite its effectiveness in these other skin conditions, it was never proven to work for wrinkles.

The way 5-FU works is by attacking damaged cells in the skin. It seeks out these cells, gobbles them up, and destroys them. Descriptively it sounds as though 5-FU is doing battle with the cells. And that's exactly what the skin looks like—the damaged cells become a red and inflamed "battleground."

An important difference between Retin-A and 5-FU is the way a person looks while using them. Retin-A sometimes can leave the skin red or slightly irritated. But in order to use enough 5-FU for it to work, it *must* cause bright red and crusty skin. These lesions are very noticeable and can last for weeks. Mind you, when the skin cools down, it is smoother than it was before. But on the way to smoother, it creates more havoc. It is not a pretty sight.

More often than not, 5-FU, as suggested by Dr. Milstein ten years ago, is used as an aid in the therapy of certain conditions. It may be used in conjunction with other creams for the treatment of various skin problems, including psoriasis, age spots, and warts. But there's no point in using 5-FU for wrinkles.

Most recently, attempts were made to use the drug known as interferon on skin problems. Interferon, a powerful antiviral and antitumor agent, is a naturally occurring protein. It can also be produced artificially by biotechnology. When injected into the skin, interferon can be used to treat warts, shingles, malignant melanoma, and precancerous growths, such as actinic keratoses.

Relying upon the same theory that sparked excitement over 5-FU, researchers at the University of Arizona used interferon in gel form to wipe out precancerous growths on the skin. Their results were published in the May 1990 issue of the *Journal of Dermatology and Surgical Oncology*. They showed that interferon gel worked no better than the placebo on actinic keratoses. The authors surmised that the interferon just did not penetrate well enough into the skin to do any good.

Will interferon be able to be developed into the antiwrinkle cream of the future? Anything is possible, but interferon is off to a less than auspicious start.

Techniques and Procedures

Wrinkles and acne scarring, tattoos, leg "spider" veins, facial blood vessels, sagging eyelids, excess body fat, and torn earlobes are all brought to the doctor's office for help. Removing them, diminishing their effect, or repairing them can improve your appearance as well as your self-esteem. This section will have a look at the various techniques and procedures the field of medicine has developed and used with these problems—their advantages, their limitations, and what you can expect of them.

Injectable Collagen and Other Filler Substances

In the early 1970s medical researchers began experimenting with a new idea. They hoped to use collagen from animals and put it into human skin. Collagen is a part of the second layer of the skin, or the dermis. To a great degree, the firmness of the skin depends upon collagen. As it decreases, wrinkles and sagging result. So, by extracting collagen from animals, these scientists were looking for a way to beef up human skin, literally and figuratively!

Over a number of years a method of purifying bovine (cow's) collagen had been perfected. This resulted in a product that could be injected underneath people's skin with only a small chance of rejection. The injected collagen replaces the worn-out human collagen, giving the skin a new lease on life.

Injected collagen allowed deep wrinkles to be erased or re-markably improved. Pitted acne scars can be lifted up by injecting collagen underneath them. In just a few short years, a major cosmetic breakthrough had come about.

The product, called Zyderm, was marketed by the Collagen Corporation of Palo Alto, California. Zyderm was approved for medical use in 1981. Since then over three hundred fifty thousand people have received close to five million injections.

| Since 1981 over 350,000 people have received collagen injections. |

However, not everyone is a good candidate for collagen injections. People who suffer from the collagen vascular diseases such as lupus are discouraged from using this treatment. There is fear that for people with these autoimmune system diseases, the foreign collagen may trigger an immune system reaction that could damage the body's tolerance of its own collagen.

But even if you are free of autoimmune disease you must first be tested for allergies to this product. A test site on the forearm is selected. Then a small amount of collagen is injected under the skin. The skin is evaluated at forty-eight hours and again in four weeks. If any redness or swelling occurs, the person is deemed allergic. Some physicians like to do a repeat test again after one month, just to be sure.

If all goes well with the testing, the treatment can proceed. Every physician who uses it develops a personal technique of injecting. Most commonly the serial injection technique is used for wrinkles. Instead of injecting a large amount of collagen all at once, a series of injections is used along the length of the wrinkle. This serves to lift up the wrinkle and flatten it out. The Collagen Corporation encourages overcorrection of the wrinkle—injecting the collagen until the wrinkled area begins to swell up. The excess material is absorbed over the next few days and the desired smooth skin look results.

The same basic technique is employed for the treatment of acne scars. The scars that respond the best are the rounded, sloping scars. Sharp and deep scars, referred to as ice pick scars, do not do well with collagen. They must be cut out, dermabraded (see below), or lasered.

Several years ago, two new collagen products were introduced. Zyderm II is a more concentrated version of the original product. It is useful for somewhat deeper scars. Zyplast is the latest of the collagen injectables. It is meant for the treatment of very deep defects, such as traumatic scars or deep furrows caused by wrinkles.

Immediately after the injections, the areas will look red and swollen, but this improves dramatically over the next day or two. Unlike some of the more involved cosmetic procedures, with collagen injections you can actually go out in public within twenty-four hours.

Collagen is also used in combination with—frequently after—other procedures, like chemical peels or face lifts (discussed below). Peels or face lifts will generally remove most of the wrinkles but can leave some stragglers. Those are the ones best treated subsequently by collagen injections. Zyderm works especially well for wrinkles around the mouth. These are especially a problem when women use lipstick, for it can seep into these wrinkles, making them even more obvious and unsightly. Collagen does a good job of flattening them out.

The effects of collagen injections only last from six months to one year.

However, the biggest shortcoming of collagen injections is that their effects only last from six months to one year. Then, new collagen must be injected. Zyplast lasts longer than Zyderm because it is a thicker compound and is injected deeper into the skin.

Another problem with collagen injections is quite uncommon but very bothersome. Allergies to it can develop down the line after using it on several occasions. Why this happens is unknown. The allergy tends to manifest itself as tender bumps at the points of injection. These can last for two to four months before they subside on their own. Fortunately this doesn't happen often. There have been several women who have had collagen injections and have claimed that they developed collagen vascular diseases, such as dermatomyositis, as a result of the injections. Although none of the subsequent lawsuits brought by these women has prevailed in court, the Collagen Corporation keeps a close watch on such allegations and investigates them thoroughly.

A newer filler substance that was introduced in the past few years is called Fibrel. It works well for scars and wrinkles of all kinds. Basically, it works the same as collagen although its composition is different. It is a mixture composed of blood that has been drawn from the person who is to be treated with it. To this is added a gelatin powder along with a substance called epsilon-aminocaproic acid. Fibrel does tend to be associated with stronger reactions than Zyderm. Thus, a swollen spot may result around the injected area that can last for days to weeks. However, on the plus side, Fibrel tends to last longer than Zyderm. Also, many experts maintain that Fibrel is more effective for deeper scars than Zyderm is.

Since long-term follow-up studies on Fibrel are lacking, it is difficult to assess what results can be expected over the years. At this point, Fibrel seems to be a wonderful alternative for those who are allergic to collagen, but the collagen vs. Fibrel debate will no doubt continue for a few more years.

Finally, we must go "back to the future" for a look at another filler product. When injectable silicone was first introduced over thirty years ago, it was touted as a miracle product for cosmetic injections and surgery. Instead, it proved to be a disaster. A number of people developed allergic reactions that resulted in permanent disfigurement. And, unlike collagen, silicone does not dissolve or get broken down. It remains in its original form permanently, as silicone. As a result of this, it was removed from the market and forgotten for two decades.

> **Most likely, the FDA will not give approval to silicone injections unless very careful, long-term studies demonstrate conclusively that they are safe and effective.**

Recent interest in injectable filler substances has given some researchers the impetus to take a second look at silicone. Indeed, the fact that silicone has a permanent effect is desirable for the treatment of scars that need to be reinjected often—both time and money are saved. However, one drawback with permanency is that while the skin changes with age, the lump of injected silicone stays the same. So, for example, over time the silicone may stand out and create an unnatural look. However, many physicians feel it has its place, and they would like to see silicone reintroduced to the market with tighter restrictions. Most likely, the FDA will not give it approval unless very careful, long-term studies demonstrate conclusively that silicone injections are safe and effective.

All these various injectable filler substances give people a chance at a new look. Frown lines, smile lines, whistle marks, and acne scars are just a few of the facial lines and marks that can be corrected.

Chemical Peels

A chemical peel is one among several ways to rejuvenate the skin. Although the art of chemical peeling is quite old, newer chemicals and refined techniques have generated a good deal of excitement in this field.

The basic concept of chemical peeling is very simple. An acid is applied to the skin in order to remove certain layers. There can be variation in the number of layers removed and also in the size of the area that is peeled away. Large areas of the face can be treated this way, or spot peels can be employed for a single trouble spot.

Peels work by removing those layers of the skin that contain the imperfection that bothers the patient. The removal process involves techniques that in a controlled way actually wound the skin at the site of the imperfection. This then "invites" the healing process to take place, which involves generating new skin cells to replace the wounded ones. The product of this healing process is a new, smooth layer of skin. The face is an ideal place for this to take place because the face has a relatively high number of pilosebaceous units—hair follicle and oil gland units—which are so helpful in regenerating new skin. Although the face is far and away the most common site peeled, the neck and hands can be peeled as well.

Quite a few cosmetic problems on the face can be improved with a chemical peel. And, as one might expect, the deeper the peel, the more the improvement. Fine wrinkles can be eliminated and deep wrinkles can be remarkably improved. In fact, the results are often dramatic. Age spots are another favorite target of peeling. These can either be treated by the spot peel method or as part of a full face peel. Active acne, as mentioned earlier, can be helped by a series of applications of weaker peels. Superficial acne scarring can be improved by the

> With a chemical peel, fine wrinkles can be eliminated and deep wrinkles can be remarkably improved.

stronger peels. Deep pitted acne scars, however, usually require other methods, such as dermabrasion (discussed below) or excision (cutting out a scar and stitching up the remaining defect). Scaly, sun-damaged spots, known as keratoses, can also be improved by this method.

Trichloroacetic acid is the most commonly used agent for chemical peels. It can be used in varying strengths from very weak to very strong. Weaker peels are generally used for the treatment of acne. Medium strength peels can be used for a freshening effect on the face. These medium strength peels can also be used on the neck and back of the hands.

The strongest and thus deepest peels with this acid are used for moderate wrinkles and acne scarring. These peels, unlike the weaker ones, are often occluded—that is, tape is applied to the entire face after the acid is applied. The tape mask is removed twenty-four to forty-eight hours later.

Another peeling agent that has gained popularity is phenol. Phenol peels are only used for full-strength peeling. As in the case of the trichloracetic acid, phenol peels can either be occluded or unoccluded. Phenol peels can usually penetrate deeper than trichloroacetic acid peels and, therefore, they can remove deeper wrinkles. On the other hand, as a result of deeper penetration, phenol peels tend to knock out more of the pigment-producing melanocytes. This can leave the skin with somewhat of a "whited out" look that may not resolve with time.

The AHAs, as discussed earlier, are not only used in their weaker strengths as home topical treatments for wrinkles, age spots, dry skin, and acne; in their much stronger strengths they are used for minipeels. These, in fact, are the newest group of peeling agents to come onto the scene. The AHA that is most widely used for this purpose is glycolic acid. It tends to be a weaker agent than trichloroacetic acid or phenol and, as such, lends itself to more frequent application.

Complications and Side Effects of Chemical Peels

As with any cosmetic procedure, complications that result from chemical peels are possible. The most potential for ominous complications occur in relation to phenol peels. Phenol is a strong substance that can be rapidly absorbed into the body. If too much phenol is applied to the face too quickly, heart irregularities can result. Different types of arrhythmias can occur. Before physicians knew of the toxic effects of phenol, several deaths resulted from its use. Thus, the usual phenol peel is now carried out slowly over a period of one to three hours to prevent too rapid an absorption. However, trichloroacetic acid and the AHAs have no systemic toxicity and have never been associated with any deaths.

As a general rule, the deeper the peel, the more pain is involved. Phenol peels are the most painful. Since most people undergoing a phenol peel are hooked up to an intravenous line just in case a complication occurs, the pain medication is often administered intravenously. Many people are also given medication to take

> **As a general rule, the deeper the peel, the more pain is involved.**

prior to the procedure. This is administered either orally or intra-muscularly.

Irregularly shaped patches of skin of different shades or hues are the most frequent complications of chemical peels. Although they are almost always temporary, they can last up to six months after the procedure is performed. The closer your natural skin tone is to an olive color, the more risk there is for this temporary blotch-iness. Some experts maintain that trichloroacetic acid peels are the most likely to lead to brownish patches. These irregular patches of pigmentation almost never occur in fair-skinned individuals, like blue-eyed blondes. Hypopigmentation, or diminished colora-tion, tends to occur with the phenol peels in certain areas, as was mentioned earlier, although some hypopigmentation can be seen in trichloroacetic acid peels as well.

Herpes simplex, the skin virus that causes fever blisters (cold sores) may be activated as a result of having a face peel. Even with prophylactic therapy, the blisters may still break through. The episodes

Fever blisters may be activated as a result of having a face peel.

are, however, usually mild and resolve spontaneously. Scarring is a rare complication of chemical peels. It has been estimated that the incidence of scarring from chemical peels is one out of every ten thousand people.

For reasons that are not well understood, firm, linear bands of thickened skin may occur on any area of the face. These bands are small. Many resolve by themselves without any treatment. The areas around the mouth and jawline appear to be the most commonly affected.

Despite the fact that the face is quite raw in appearance for the first few days after a peel, there is a remarkably low rate of infection, although topical and/or oral antibiotics are generally used prophylactically. Proper postpeel care is essential in promot-ing wound healing. This includes changing dressings, avoiding the sun, and other practices that are commonly followed to help with wound healing.

Which peel type is right for you? This is something you should determine together with your physician. Consideration should be given to several factors: What do you want to accomplish? What skin type do you have? How prone are you to develop pigment changes? How much time are you willing to be or can you accom-modate being out of the public eye? Do you have a tendency to-wards scarring?

Chemical peels offer an advantage over face lifts (discussed below) in several respects. They are usually less costly and carry less of a risk. In addition, while face lifts are effective for deep wrinkles and sagging, they do nothing for the color and brightness of the skin itself. Even light peels make a distinct improvement in skin tone and texture. When done properly, chemical peels can really improve the quality of your skin. On the other hand, chemical peels do not achieve the success in treating the deeper problems that face lifts tackle.

Dermabrasion

Dermabrasion is just what it sounds like—abrasion of the dermis, or skin. It involves mechanically planing down the skin to give it a smoother yet natural look. This is accomplished by using a high-speed rotating wheel that abrades (rubs away or wears down) the skin surface down to the depth necessary to get rid of the problem being treated. A number of different wheels are available to the cosmetic surgeon, depending on the skin problem to be treated. Wheels with wire brushes, diamond fraises, or serrated metal edges are available. Each physician develops a feel for which wheel to use and when. Not only do the wheels differ in the surface they abrade with, they differ in size. Larger ones are used for broader areas and smaller ones are used for spots that require a finer touch. They are hand-held units that are powered by electricity or by compressed nitrogen gas. Depending upon the unit used, the wheel can spin anywhere from four hundred RPM to sixty thousand RPM.

Before abrading the skin, the physician must first anesthetize it. Most of the time, this is accomplished by spraying a topical anesthetic on the area to be treated. This freezes the skin for about thirty seconds. While the skin is frozen, the dermabrasion is carried out. An alternative to freezing is to inject anesthetic into key points on the face where the facial nerves run. Regardless of the mode used for local anesthetizing, some people who get a dermabrasion receive an intramuscular injection of a strong pain reliever prior to the procedure. This can be augmented by oral and/or intravenous medications as well, depending upon the person's pain tolerance.

Dermabrasion is used most commonly in the treatment of acne scarring. Chemical peels have already been discussed for treating acne scarring, but they are effective mainly for superficial scars. The severe inflammation associated with some types of acne leaves pits or holes in the face. For this deep acne scarring, which is often widespread across the face, dermabrasion is often *the* treatment of choice. (Unfortunately, acne scarring on the back does not lend itself to treatment with dermabrasion. The skin on the back is different from facial skin, with the result that dermabrasion performed on the back has a very marked tendency to produce scarring that is uglier than the acne scars themselves.) For deep scarring more than one dermabrasion is often required in order to attempt to correct the problem. Two, three, or four dermabrasions may be necessary in severe cases. The intervals between the treatments can be from six to twelve months, until the doctor and patient feel that the desired result is achieved. As in the case of chemical peels, not only are the old scars improved, but if there is any active acne it often gets better as a result of the dermabrasion.

> **For deep scarring more than one dermabrasion is often required.**

In addition to using dermabrasion for acne scarring, many dermatologic surgeons advocate its early use on traumatic scars. Facial scars that result from an automobile accident or an assault are often irregular or jagged in their appearance. Dermabrasion can help blend such scars into their background, with the best results achieved if the dermabrasion is carried out within the first two months of the accident.

Before the advent of laser therapy, dermabrasion was the main treatment for tattoos. As with the treatment of acne scarring, in tattoo removal, the skin is abraded down to the desired level to remove as much tattoo pigment (or ink) as possible. More than one treatment may be necessary. One major difference between treating scarring and removing tattoos is that when dermabrasion is used for scarring it is carried out on the face almost exclusively, whereas tattoos can be dermabraded virtually anywhere on the body. Dermabrasion used for scarring goes much deeper, while the dermabrasion used for removing tattoos is more superficial. The deeper method only works well on the face, because the face has a much lower potential for scarring than other areas of the body. The trunk and upper arms, which have the worst scarring potential, can't benefit from deep dermabrasion because new scars will result. But tattoo dermabrasion is another story. Because it needn't be so deep, it can be used on the trunk and legs as well as the face. However, nowadays, the newer laser techniques give better results than dermabrasion in the treatment of tattoos.

A skin problem known as the rhinophyma lends itself nicely to dermabrasion. This is the big, red, bulbous nose that W. C. Fields made famous. Rhinophyma can be due to rosacea (see chapter 3) or to hereditary factors. Ingestion of alcohol makes the nose redder. Oftentimes, it can become grossly overgrown and appears almost double its normal size. Dermabrasion planes down the excessive oil glands, blood vessels, and pockets of pus that make up a rhinophyma. The results from the treatment can be amazing. A relatively normal nose can be formed from the previously very disfigured one.

Dermabrasion is also used to treat wrinkles, age spots, and superficial precancerous lesions on the face. Dermabrasion is often used for wrinkles around the mouth because precise control can be achieved in this delicate area by using this technique. However, for around the eyes, chemical peels are the treatment of choice. Dermabrasion could cause potential complications around the eyes by tearing at the skin. Sometimes a dermabrasion is used after a face lift (discussed below) in order to "fine tune" any wrinkles that might be left. But whether used in conjunction with a face lift or alone, dermabrasion can be very effective for wrinkles around the mouth. When deciding between a dermabrasion and a chemical peel one thing you will want to know is that chemical peels can be taped over or left open, while dermabrasions are almost always taped and covered. Crusts can remain for up to two weeks after the dermabrasion is performed. The same skin care plan and avoidance of sun is recommended as is recommended with chemical peels.

The Complications and Side Effects of Dermabrasion

Dermabrasion, like almost any other cosmetic procedure, is not utterly without complications and side effects. Fortunately, they are uncommon, but anyone contemplating a dermabrasion should be made aware of them.

The most common side effect is the formation of multiple milia, or whiteheads. There are many theories as to why these whiteheads develop, but no one knows for sure. However, they will disappear on their own within one year.

Around the jawline there is a tendency for what is known as hypertrophic scarring. These are somewhat

Dermabrasion's most common side effect is whiteheads, but facial scars and changes in pigmentation can also occur.

overgrown scars that are raised over the surface of the skin. Why this particular area of the face is prone to hypertrophic scarring while other areas aren't is not known. What we do know is that the skin reacts differently on different parts of the face. Hypertrophic scarring can be treated with injections of cortisone or the application of cortisone creams or tape to the affected area. Another unwanted effect of dermabrasion that can occur is depressed scarring or grooving. This is generally thought to be the result of over-dermabrasion. Sometimes these grooves correct themselves, while other times the area around them needs to be re-dermabraded to get rid of them. Although not from the dermabrasion itself, a somewhat irregular type of scarring can result from overfreezing the skin with the anesthetic agent. This is essentially frostbite. Usually, however, the scarring is very mild.

As with chemical peels, there can be color changes with dermabrasion. Generally, it is loss of pigmentation rather than increased pigmentation. This is due to the destruction of the melanocytes (the pigment-producing cells) that occurs during the process of planing down the skin. Also, overaggressive freezing may destroy the melanocytes. Patchy hyperpigmentation, or excess coloration of the skin, can also occur but usually only in people with darker skin and in those who spend too much time in the sun during the first months after receiving a dermabrasion. Fortunately, hyperpigmentation tends to fade out during the six-month period following dermabrasion.

However, because these potential side effects and complications are uncommon, dermabrasion remains a very valuable and viable tool in correcting acne scarring.

The Face Lift

About fifty thousand face lifts are performed in the United States each year. Of all the cosmetic procedures described in this book, the face lift is one of the most complicated. As the name suggests, it serves the purpose of lifting up the sagging skin of the face to give a more youthful appearance.

Not everyone is a good candidate for a face lift. People who have bleeding problems or take anticoagulants should not undergo the procedure. Certain medications, such as aspirin or birth control pills, should be avoided for two to three weeks before the surgery.

And surgery it is. Several incisions have to be made on the face and scalp, followed by an extensive process of pulling the facial skin tighter. General anesthesia is usually necessary.

The basic technique of a face lift is to separate the skin structure from the muscle that lies beneath it. This is called "undermining." Once the skin has been freed up, it can then be pulled tighter.

In order to be able to undermine the skin, several incisions must first be made on the face and scalp. Every cosmetic surgeon favors certain techniques over others. A common method is to cut the skin from the hairline near the temples down across the front part of the ear. The incision is then carried behind the ear onto the back of the scalp. Incisions are then placed in areas of the face where they will be least visible. Once these incisions have been made, surgical instruments are used to separate the tissues. The separation is carried out from the ears all the way to the nose. Extreme caution must be taken not to cut any nerves or arteries. When the skin is finally pulled tighter, it is stitched in place, and the excess skin is removed.

> For a face lift, several incisions have to be made, followed by an extensive process of pulling the facial skin tighter.

Once the operation is complete, the face and scalp are wrapped up like a mummy to insure that everything stays in place. Despite the tight wrappings, the person can still eat and breathe. Most of the sutures are removed within a week. Pain may continue for days to weeks after the surgery.

Side Effects and Complications of Face Lifts

As you can imagine, several potential side effects and complications may arise from having a face lift done. The most common problem is the formation of a hematoma—a collection of blood underneath the skin. This can occur from the severing of blood vessels that takes place in the process of separating tissues. Despite the best efforts to stop the resultant bleeding that may occur, hematomas can develop. In fact, this complication is seen in about 10 percent of those women who undergo a face lift. Often, the hematomas can be eliminated by nicking the skin with a blade or by suctioning them out with a needle. The sooner they are removed, the better. The longer they remain, the greater the likelihood of their distorting the contour of the skin or causing infection.

> A hematoma—a collection of blood underneath the skin—occurs in about 10 percent of those who undergo a face lift.

Sloughing, or shedding, of the skin happens in about one out of twenty women who have this procedure. Sloughing occurs when the blood supply to a portion of the skin gets choked off, causing that portion of the skin to die. Several things can lead to it—the severance of an artery, an underlying hematoma, or skin that is too tight. Unfortunately, once the skin begins to slough, there is nothing that can be done except to hope that the scar it leaves is not very noticeable.

Another undesirable effect of the skin having been pulled too tight is hair loss in the area above and in front of the ears. This hair loss can be permanent. Also, just as arteries can be cut, so can nerves. This usually leads to numbness on the affected side of the face where the nerves were damaged. And the numbness can last for several months! On rare occasions it can be permanent. When the nerves that are cut are ones that control muscle movement, a drooping, or paralysis, can occur. Although all of these are unusual complications, it is important that you know they are possible.

Liposuction, which is discussed immediately below, is sometimes used to fine-tune a face lift by removing fat deposits left behind. This is frequently done during the actual face lift itself. Actually, several similarities exist between liposuction and face lifting. Both involve making incisions in the skin in order to go deep into the tissues. Both are associated with postoperative pain and numbness. And both have a high rate of success.

Specific Attributes and Limitations of the Face Lift

As was stated earlier, face lifts can remove deep wrinkles and shore up sagging skin. However, unlike peels and dermabrasion the face lift does nothing for skin complexion. Also, it may not remove fine wrinkling around the mouth. For these reasons a face lift is sometimes followed by a face peel or dermabrasion.

Although face lifts can make a remarkable difference in your appearance, the forces of nature eventually get the upper hand. With time, the skin begins to sag back down again and the wrinkles return. Face lifts commonly need to be repeated every five to ten years. Fortunately, most women who have already had one face lift say that the second time around is more tolerable than the first. No, a face lift isn't fun, but it does get easier.

Face lifts commonly need to be repeated every five to ten years.

Liposuction

Liposuction involves the suctioning of fat out of the body. Cosmetic surgeons who perform liposuction use a long, hollow, metal tube called a cannula. Cannulas come in different sizes and shapes to allow surgeons to remove fat from different parts of the body. Longer ones are used for fat around the thighs and abdomen, while shorter ones are more in vogue for facial work. Some cannulas are curved. The cannulas are connected to a special vacuum that sucks out the fat particles that have been loosened up. Most recently, several cosmetic surgeons have advocated using a large syringe with a cannula on the end to remove the fat.

When performing this procedure, some physicians use a general anesthetic while others use only local anesthesia. Certain doctors prefer to have their patients completely knocked out by the anesthesia so that they feel no pain. Others choose to give a series of local numbing shots so that their patients can be awake during the procedure. The patient who is not asleep is able to respond to requests to change positions, which can sometimes be of help in the procedure. But either way—awake or asleep—is perfectly acceptable.

The liposuction starts with an incision in the skin. The cut is usually very small—just big enough for the cannula to fit in. The cannula is then pushed into the fatty layer of the body. When in place, the cannula is pushed back and forth. This serves to break up the fatty tissue. At the same time that the fat is being broken up, it is being sucked out of the body by the vacuum. An expert cosmetic surgeon can make a very good estimate as to how much fat to remove to achieve the desired effect.

Along with the fat, a certain amount of blood and body fluids will be removed. The area that has just been treated is taped heavily. This prevents further bleeding and helps give a firm and natural contour to the skin. The tape is removed in about a week.

Part of the question as to which anesthetic to use has to do with the issue of safety. The disadvantage of using general anesthesia is that there is always some risk of complications from general anesthesia. Potential candidates are always screened for any medical problems before general anesthesia is used. Local anesthesia offers the advantage of not having to undergo the risks of general anesthesia. Also, the local anesthesia can be done in the doctor's office, while general anesthesia is almost always done in the hospital. However, the local anesthesia method is somewhat painful while the numbing medicine is being injected.

The results of liposuction speak for themselves. This procedure, almost unknown ten years ago, has achieved skyrocketing popularity. Hips can be smoothed, abdomens can be flattened, double chins become single again. The number one area that women request having done is the hip/buttock area. Fat can be removed from any part of the body, including behind the knee, above the knee, and on the leg. Liposuction can also be performed on select areas of the face, such as the cheeks or jowls. However, small scars may occur at the site where the incision was made.

How long do these results of this procedure last? That's a good question. Since liposuction is still in its infancy, we do not have any long-term follow-up studies. But the fat does seem to stay away for at least a few years. Does fat regrow faster in the buttocks than under the chin? Another good question. Only time will answer that one.

Side Effects of Liposuction

As with all cosmetic procedures, liposuction has its share of potential problems or side effects. Everyone will experience bruising and soreness in the treated areas. This may last for days or weeks. Postoperative pain ranges from bothersome to severe. Bleeding is an infrequent problem. As we mentioned before, the back and forth action of the cannula removes the fat, but it can irritate or cut small nerves as well. This leads to a temporary numbing sensation over the affected area that can last for a few months! With time, these do resolve on their own.

> With liposuction a temporary numbing sensation occurs over the affected area, and it can last for a few months!

One of the side effects that can result from this procedure is an unevenness in appearance. One hip may look like it had more fat removed than the other. This may correct itself when the swelling resolves over the next few weeks. If not, a small touchup job may be necessary. Sometimes the procedure results in a dimpling or puckering effect, giving the area worked on a wavy surface instead of a smooth one. As with the other complications, time is the best medicine. Almost all of the waviness goes away within a year or so.

Very rarely, an absolute horror story unfolds. One case involved a woman who went into the hospital for an abdominal reduction. Apparently during the liposuction, the cannula was poked too deeply into the abdomen. This created a hole in the muscle wall, which resulted in disastrous complications, resulting in death. Nightmares like these make for headlines in news magazines, but they are exceedingly rare.

Specific Cosmetic Problems and Their Treatment

Wrinkles and Acne Scarring

The anatomical differences between wrinkles and acne scars are that wrinkles result from a degradation of the underlying collagen in the skin and are usually soft and pliable, whereas acne pits are punched-out areas of skin that are the result of inflammation, and they tend to be tough and nonpliable. Yet despite their differences they are treated similarly, using one or another of two approaches: either the healthy skin is smoothed down to the lower level of the scar or wrinkle *or* the depression is lifted up to the higher level. Retin-A and the AHAs help to a certain degree with the milder scarring and more superficial wrinkles, but when these problems are deeper, more powerful methods are needed. The smoothing down process can be accomplished by chemical peels, dermabrasion, laserabrasion (described below), or face lifts.

Tattoos

Tattoos aren't just for Marines anymore. Almost half of those who get tattoos today are civilian and female. Famous film stars like Cher and Julia Roberts are among the newer aficionados. As opposed to the so-called jailhouse tattoos of yesteryear, today's tattoos are more varied in design and brighter in color. Because of their increased popularity, several magazines dedicated solely to the practice of self-decoration have emerged.

> Many who get tattoos eventually want them removed—over 50 percent by some estimates.

Yet, however much tattoos have increased in popularity with newer groups of people, the fact remains that many who get tattoos eventually want them removed—over 50 percent by some estimates. The reasons are many, only one of which is that it is not usually very appealing to most people to have the name of someone who is no longer your true love emblazoned on your body. Besides tattoos that name a current love, there are gang-related tattoos. In fact, being tattooed with the name of your gang or group can be part of its initiation rites, or it can be a way to show you are "cool." Sometimes being tattooed with your nickname serves a similar social function.

Certain ethnic groups have dots tattooed onto their cheeks, chin, or fingers. Some people have designs tattooed; some choose initials. A common tattoo pattern is to have the letters *L-O-V-E* tattooed onto the top of the fingers. And, yes, people still get tattoos done while they are inebriated, only to wake up in the morning with a rude reminder of the night before.

So much for the social dimension of tattooing. At the physical level tattoos are pigmented particles that are burned deep into the dermis. As such, they are permanently placed into the skin. Like any other foreign substance, the body can develop an allergic reaction to tattoo pigments. Most often it is the red dye that gives an allergic or granulomatous response. These are itchy, deep bumps at the site of the tattoo injection, which may be treated with either excision or injections of corticosteroids into the affected areas.

> Itchy, deep bumps at the site of the tattoo injection are signs of an allergic reaction to tattoo pigments.

It is a cosmetic surgical challenge to remove a tattoo and leave as little scarring as possible. Several options exist. One is the elliptical excision. This is used on linear tattoos, where the tattoo consists of lettering, as with a name or word. This technique involves the cutting out of an oval piece of skin surrounding the tattoo and then closing the wound with stitches. This results in a linear scar in place of the tattoo. Some tattoos are too large or their location makes it too difficult to use an elliptical excision as a method of removal. For these, the tattoo is excised and instead of stitching the wound as described above, a skin graft is placed over the wound because it is too large to be stitched. The disadvantage of skin grafting is that the grafted skin rarely matches the surrounding skin, and the place on the body from which the skin is taken is also scarred.

Dermabrasion is another useful technique for removing tattoos. As is done with acne scars, the skin is sanded down to the lowest level of what is to be removed, in this case, the tattoo pigment, and then left to heal in. However, most tattoos are not on the face, where dermabrasion works best because of the many oil glands and hair follicles that help normal skin regenerate more easily. Because other parts of the body, such as the arms and back, do not heal as elegantly in response to deep abrasions, when this technique is used on them there is always the possibility of hypertrophic, or overactive, scarring.

Yes, there are techniques to minimize scarring, but the physician walks a tightrope between getting out as much pigment as possible and trying to avoid hypertrophic scarring. One technique that is helpful is called salabrasion, a variation on standard dermabrasion in which the skin is abraded down to the level of the tattoo pigment and then treated with an acid for several days. This lifts out the pigment but spares as much normal tissue as possible. However, no matter how perfectly the abrasion is done, there is bound to be some scarring because the pigment sits too deeply in the dermis to avoid this complication.

The scar that results from a dermabraded tattoo is a light-colored patch of skin, often studded with remnant specks of the tattoo pigment that were too deep to get out. These remaining specks are usually not very noticeable, but if they are, they can be dermabraded a second time. Cosmetic surgeons take great pains to make the scar assume a pattern that does not reflect the exact outline of the tattoo but instead has an oval or rounded shape. This is done to avoid drawing attention to the area that would otherwise stand out if it assumed a square or sharply defined configuration.

The CO_2 laser can be used to laserabrade the tattoo in a manner similar to dermabrasion. Whereas dermabrasion is performed on skin that is frozen with a spray, a local anesthesia is injected for a laserabrasion. Salabrasion can be combined with laserabrasion. Some experts argue that laserabrasion offers finer control and therefore a better cosmetic result than dermabrasion.

Another type of laser, the Q-switched ruby laser, operates on a different principle than the CO_2 laser. Instead of burning through the skin, the Q-switched ruby laser passes through the epidermis into the dermis without altering the skin itself. The laser beam is only absorbed by the tattoo particles. The particles then "explode" underneath the skin, and the fragments are gobbled up by the scavenger cells, the lymphocytes. This procedure is repeated over a series of visits un-

The Q-switched ruby laser is currently considered to be the state-of-the-art way to remove tattoos.

til all of the fragments are absorbed. The advantage of this technique is that the skin is not broken, and thus hypertrophic scarring is eliminated and discoloration is minimized. The downside is that three to seven treatment sessions are necessary, and pigment can remain. The Q-switched ruby laser is much more effective on amateur, blue ink tattoos than on professional, multicolored ones. It is currently considered to be the state-of-the-art way to remove tattoos. The Q-switched YAG laser operates on the same principle.

Obviously, there is room for improvement in all of the techniques used for tattoo removal. But I must say that despite the minor drawbacks, virtually 100 percent of the people whom I have treated for tattoo removal, by whatever technique, are satisfied with the results. Perhaps it is the relief at never having to see the tattoo again. But, whatever the reason, most tattoo removals are well-accepted.

Questions and Answers

Q. *I've heard that tattoos will completely fade out with time. Is that true?*

A. Not true at all. Once the tattoo pigment is placed into the skin, it stays there until it is removed.

Q. *Does laserabrasion work better than dermabrasion for tattoo removal?*

A. It depends on the skill of the physician. Some like one technique, others like the other.

Q. *If someone has a laser treatment, can they develop cancer from it twenty years later?*

A. No. There has never been any evidence linking laser surgery with any cancer risk.

Q. *How long does it take for a CO_2 lasered spot to heal?*

A. It can take up to a month depending upon what type of acid you use. Without any acid use, it takes about two weeks.
There will be a persistent redness for up to six months, which will fade with time into a lighter pink-white color.

Q. *Does the Q-switched ruby laser treatment require any anesthesia?*

A. No. It stings a bit while it is being performed, but no anesthesia is necessary.

Varicose Veins

Every woman will develop some degree of varicose veins during her lifetime. They are more common in women who have had one or more children and in those whose work keeps them on their feet all day. The constant pressure on the leg veins causes them to swell. Then, once the walls of the blood vessels have been stretched, they remain distended.

> Varicose veins are more common in women who have had one or more children and in those whose work keeps them on their feet all day.

Varicose veins may vary in size from a fraction of a millimeter to more than a centimeter. Although they are a cosmetic problem, they can also sometimes be painful. And, for the larger vessels, there exists the possibility of blood clot formation.

Injecting a solution into superficial varicose (spider) veins is a very old practice, one that is more art than science. It is called sclerotherapy and is also used on the larger varicose veins. But not all varicose veins are amenable to sclerotherapy. Some of the tinier varicose veins are too small to inject—even with the smallest of needles. And the extra large blood vessels are best treated with vein stripping, an extensive surgical procedure that requires hospitalization.

The basic concept of sclerotherapy is quite simple. Using the appropriate size needle—several different needle sizes are available to the physician and the choice depends on upon the size of the blood vessel—a solution is injected into the dilated veins. The solution irritates the inner walls of the blood vessels and causes them to constrict and collapse inward. This is called shrinking. It makes the veins invisible.

Several different injectable solutions—called sclerosing solutions or sclerosants—can be used. The most commonly employed sclerosant is a simple salt solution. In fact, sodium chloride in various concentrations is currently the favorite injectable solution used in sclerotherapy. Other chemicals, such as sodium sotradechol, aethoxysklerol, and concentrated sugar solutions, are available as well. Each one has its own pluses and minuses, but all are considered safe. Exactly how the sclerosing solution works is not clearly understood. Most investigators agree that the inside of the blood vessel wall becomes irritated by the solution and clamps down on itself, thereby shutting off the blood supply. Others believe that a tiny blood clot is formed, which gradually resolves over the next few weeks leaving a nonworking blood vessel. Whatever the mechanism, it works.

The technique of injecting varicose veins requires a steady hand and a sharp eye. The fine needle is poked through the overlying skin and threaded into the vein. The solution is then injected. If a central vein is chosen, one that feeds other smaller veins, a remarkable phenomenon then occurs. The central vein and all of its feeder vessels blanch out (turn white) when the sclerosing solution travels through them. This produces a sensation that can range from a mild tingle to a burning flush. Pressure is usually applied immediately afterwards in order to keep the veins compressed. Tightly wrapped adhesive tape is often applied. At the same office visit, the physician continues to treat the other veins in a similar manner.

Sclerotherapy can be backbreaking work for the doctor! Good lighting, a cooperative patient, and good nursing assistance are all important. Usually, the physician will single out a particular segment for that first day's session—for example, doing only one leg or only one thigh or simply setting a time limit of fifteen to twenty minutes to do whatever can be done in that period. Treatments can be repeated monthly. It may take from one to eight sessions, depending on the response to each treatment and on the number of blood vessels involved.

And, not to worry, the superficial varicose veins are not needed to maintain normal blood circulation in the leg and thighs. Therefore, eliminating them with sclerotherapy carries no danger of choking off the essential blood supply to those areas.

The Side Effects of Sclerotherapy

Although they are usually minor, there are some untoward effects that can occur with sclerotherapy. Almost everyone will experience a temporary black-and-blue effect around the injected veins. This is due to the displacement of the blood from the vein when the solution is injected. This will resolve with a month's time. However, up to a third of people who undergo sclerotherapy will develop brown spots that can last from six to eighteen months. About 5 percent will maintain these brown spots for more than two years. For those whose spots do not fade, a bleaching chemical, similar to those used in chemical peels, is applied in order to lighten the color. Originally it was thought

> **Almost everyone will experience a temporary black-and-blue effect around the injected varicose veins.**

that the brown color was due to melanin, the skin pigment. Lately, it has been determined that the spots are due to hemosiderin, a breakdown product of blood that assumes a brownish tinge.

A problem that occurs in about 3 percent of the people treated for varicose veins is swelling of the ankles. This is more common in those who have a previous history of leg swelling. It is also more likely to occur when large amounts of sclerosing solution are injected during a single session. This swelling goes down over the next few days without any other problems.

When larger veins are treated, the possibility of creating a small blood clot exists. This blood clot, referred to as thrombophlebitis, is seen in less than 1 percent of sclerotherapy recipients. Treatments of this side effect consist of aspirin or another similar anti-inflammation medication. Antibiotics, compression, and heat are all helpful, too.

Rarely, a small ulcer can form where the sclerosing solution was injected. This is due to irritation of the skin that lies above the varicose veins. The skin breaks down and leaves a crust. When the crust finally falls off a few weeks later, it heals with a small white scar. The scar fades out with time, but some people endure a permanent spot.

Although the above list might sound scary, in reality complications are uncommon. The satisfaction rate among women who have had sclerotherapy runs over 90 percent.

Questions and Answers

Q. *Does pregnancy cause spider veins?*
A. Pregnancy is one of the leading contributing factors towards the development of spider veins. The excess weight of pregnancy bogs down the circulation.

Q. *How much improvement can I expect with sclerotherapy?*
A. Expect about 75 to 80 percent improvement. Nobody gets 100 percent results, but almost everyone who has the treatment seems to experience 75 to 80 percent improvement.

Q. *How much does it hurt?*
A. This varies with the solution used, but all will cause some sort of discomfort. Usually it is a burning sensation that has the feeling of traveling up or down the leg. As soon as the solution is withdrawn, the burning ceases. The initial needle prick it-

self causes a very slight pain because such small sized needles are used.

Q. *Can I jog or play tennis soon after the treatment?*

A. It is usually not advisable. Some physicians encourage walking after treatment while others discourage it. Most agree that
either the legs should be wrapped for several days or support
hose should be worn for two weeks.

Q. *How long does the black-and-blue color last?*

A. About two weeks. In a very small percentage of women, the
black-and-blue color will give way to a persistent light brown
speck, which can last many months. The speck fades away
with time but can be unsightly while it is present.

Q. *Can spider veins be prevented?*

A. Regular exercise, avoiding long periods of standing, and
keeping your weight down all are preventative measures.

Q. *Are deep varicose veins different than superficial spider
veins?*

A. Yes. Deep varicose veins are large and can lead to dangerous situations such as blood clot formation. The formation of
superficial spider veins does not necessarily indicate that
deeper varicose veins are present.

Facial Blood Vessels

Small blood vessels on the face can result from quite a number of
causes:

1▶ There may be a hereditary tendency to develop them.
2▶ Exposure to the sun can thin out the skin and cause blood vessels to become visible.
3▶ Pregnancy and birth control pills both provide estrogen stimulation to blood vessels, causing them to grow and become
prominent.
4▶ Certain diseases such as rosacea are associated with facial
acne and an increase in facial blood vessels.
5▶ Alcohol intake can dilate the blood vessels of the face.
6▶ Liver failure, with concomitant failure to break down estrogens, can also dilate the facial blood vessels.

Several things can be done about facial blood vessels. Makeup can be used to camouflage them. The underlying cause can be treated or eliminated so as to prevent formation of new vessels. They can be ignored. Or they can be removed.

One of the most common ways to treat facial blood vessels is to electrodesiccate them. A fine needle is placed on top of or into the vessel and an electric current is then turned on. The current runs up the blood vessel, thereby destroying it. Although this technique is usually successful, the vessels can sometimes recur. Also, if the current is too strong, a slight depression can be left at the affected area.

Sometimes, the CO_2 laser is used to "zap" a resistant blood vessel, especially when it is around the nose. Local anesthesia is necessary when using the CO_2 laser for this purpose.

Another group of lasers, sometimes referred to as the colored light lasers, can also be used for this purpose. The original in this class was the argon laser, with the more recent additions being the dye laser and the copper laser. These lasers emit a wavelength that is selectively absorbed by the blood vessels. Therefore, they pass through the epidermis without causing any damage to it. As the blood vessel pops underneath the skin, it leaves a black-and-blue mark for seven to ten days. There is no need for anesthesia, but each "zap" feels like the snap of a rubber band. Small blood vessels on the face respond better than vessels on other parts of the body to this treatment.

Larger vascular patches, such as portwine stains, can be treated with the colored light lasers as well. A portwine stain is a large red birthmark that is often found in the head and neck region. Mikhail Gorbachev has one on his forehead. One the size of his would take five or six treatments to remove. Still, about 10 percent of the color generally remains after the final treatment.

About four years ago a woman came to see me who had a portwine stain that covered the entire left side of her face, although it seemed to have been partially removed, as there were areas of white scarring. I took one look at her and said, "You had an argon laser treatment ten years ago." To which she responded that exactly nine years earlier, she indeed had an argon laser treatment. The appearance of her face had the classic look of an argon treated portwine stain—a partial clearing with areas of fine white scarring. We decided to clear up the residual portwine stain with the dye laser. After five treatments, that's exactly what happened. But the white scarring left by the previous argon laser treatment was still there, and there was not much we could do about it except to cover it with makeup.

Questions and Answers

Q. *Do any of the lasers affect pregnancy or childbirth?*

A. No, there is no systemic absorption of laser energy to affect a fetus.

Q. *Is the argon laser outdated?*

A. Although there are some very specialized uses still left for the argon laser, it has basically been supplanted by the dye laser in the treatment of facial veins.

Sagging Eyelids

Blepharoplasty is the performance of cosmetic surgery of the eyelids. Eyelid surgery is one of the most intricate cosmetic procedures around. A good deal of experience is needed to perform these operations.

There are three physical factors that can lead to a baggy eyelid: (1) *overgrown skin*—where the skin of the eyelid has become lax with time and hangs down; (2) *excess fat*—where the fat pads around the eye that help to cushion and protect it bulge out, resulting in a baggy eyelid; (3) *large eye muscles*—where the muscle that surrounds the eye, called the orbicularis oculi muscle, enlarges and pushes everything outward. However, studies have shown that people who are habitual squinters can develop eyelid bagginess as well.

A woman's eyelid differs from a man's. In men, there is a tendency for the eyebrow to hang down lower. This creates the image of the eyelids being pushed back deeper into the face. On the other hand, the upper eyelid is quite prominent in women. In fact, if you measured the distance between the eyebrow and the eyelid, women would have an advantage of several millimeters. All this might seem trivial, but they are important facts for the cosmetic surgeon to keep in mind when performing blepharoplasty. Nobody's face is 100 percent alike on both sides. The differences, although slight, are much more noticeable in the eyelid area than on other parts of the face. Thus the eyelids are seldom the same going

| Women's upper eyelids are more prominent than men's. |

into cosmetic surgery, and they may not be the same coming out. But the difference between them has to be in keeping with that person's look and what is desired. This is what makes blepharoplasty such an exacting and challenging procedure.

Blepharoplasty is the number one cosmetic surgery in Asia. There, it is performed mostly in an effort to westernize the appearance of the face by transforming the configuration of the oriental eyelid shape to that of the occidental shape.

Before a blepharoplasty is performed, the eyelids must be thoroughly evaluated. Any unevenness between the two sides has to be carefully noted in order to decide on the surgical approach to be taken. The eyelids are pinched with an instrument to see how much tissue to remove. When all of the calculations have been made, a marking pen outlines the plan of "attack."

Either general or local anesthesia may be used. Some physicians prefer local anesthesia because they may want the person to open and close the eyes during the procedure. This enables the physician to make sure that not too much or too little skin is removed.

Whether local or general anesthesia is used, once it has taken effect, the surgeon is ready to go. Delicately, the skin is cut to expose the deeper layers. The excess skin is removed. The muscle layer is the next to be reckoned with. The appropriate amount of muscle is cut out ever so gingerly. Finally, the fat layer is exposed. Using a light hand, the fat is teased out of its pouch. The necessary portion is taken out, and the surgery is almost complete. Each layer must be stitched back together to itself. Very fine sutures are used in order to minimize damage to the tissues.

The cosmetic surgeon's approach to the lower eyelid is somewhat different than it is with the upper one. Subtle differences in anatomy between the two dictate another approach. And the smaller the area, the more intricate and delicate the approach. An error of just two millimeters can make an enormous difference.

Surgery to the eyelids result in their remaining black and blue for about two weeks. Keeping the eyes at rest helps the healing process. Squinting, wide opening, and even too much reading can affect healing.

> Up to 10 percent of those who get a blepharoplasty will need a touchup treatment.

Up to 10 percent of those who get a blepharoplasty will need a touchup treatment. Most of the time it's for an uneven appearance between the two eyes. It is best to wait awhile to see how the eyelids heal before attempting to have them realigned. The most common serious side effect occurs when too much skin has been removed. When this happens, it becomes difficult for the eyelids to close completely. This problem needs to be corrected promptly. If not, damage can occur to the eyeball.

Unfortunately, as with the other cosmetic procedures, nothing lasts forever. After a few years, the eyelids may begin to sag again.

It should be noted that some of the women who may want cosmetic intervention on their eyelids are not treatable with blepharoplasty. For example, women who experience eyelid swelling during their menstrual cycles will not be helped by eyelid surgery. Also, for getting rid of fine wrinkles on the eyelids, a chemical peel would be better suited than blepharoplasty. Crow's feet—the fine lines that streak out from the sides of the eyes towards the temples—will not be helped by blepharoplasty either. As with fine wrinkles of the eyelids, chemical peeling is the best solution for this problem.

Questions and Answers

Q. *Are drooping eyelids caused by lack of sleep?*

A. Yes and no. Your eyelids can droop somewhat due to lack of sleep, but this is only a temporary phenomenon. Heredity and facial motions are the two most common factors that cause permanent drooping.

Q. *How do I prepare for the day of the operation?*

A. By getting plenty of rest. You may need to be premedicated. Some people are awake during the procedure while others are put to sleep.

Q. *Will I remember what happened during the operation?*

A. It depends on what anesthetic was used and whether or not you were put to sleep.

Q. *How soon will I notice a difference?*

A. There may be swelling for several days after the procedure, so it may take a week or two to appreciate the final results.

Excess Body Fat

We can thank the French for their innovations in the removal of body fat. They were the first to perfect the technique that came to be known as liposuction. "Lipo" means "fat," and getting rid of it is a big fat problem. (Pun intended!) Several French cosmetic surgeons hit upon the idea that fat could be broken up with a needle and then sucked out of the body. The French perfected this method over the course of several years before others started to use it.

Questions and Answers

Q. *Is it true that some people cannot metabolize the fat in their tissues as well as others?*

A. Yes. Everyone's metabolism is different, so the individual propensity to produce or reduce fat cells varies from person to person.

Q. *What is cellulite?*

A. That's a good question. Cellulite means different things to different people. In general, the medical community shies away from using the term cellulite, because it can refer to fat, to ripples in the skin, or to collagen—three different things. (And don't mistake "cellulite" for a similar word, "cellulitis," which refers to an infection of the skin, characterized by redness, swelling, and warmth.)

Q. *Does age affect whether or not I will do well with liposuction?*

A. Not really. Liposuction seems to do as well in mature age groups as it does in younger ones, although some cosmetic surgeons feel that because younger women have greater skin elasticity they make better candidates.

Q. *What are the long-term side effects of liposuction?*

A. There don't seem to be any discernible long-term side effects.

Q. *How long does it last?*

A. Months to years. Some of the remaining fat cells will regrow and renewed weight gain is always possible.

Q. *How sore will I be after liposuction?*

A. You will feel somewhat bruised and tender, but severe pain is the exception, not the rule. It might be a good idea to have someone drive you home after the procedure.

Q. *What is lipoinjection?*

A. Lipoinjection is the removal of your own fat from one location that is then injected into another fat deficient location.

The most common donor site is the buttock or thigh region. The most common recipient sites are the face and back of the hand.

Q. *How long does lipoinjection last?*

A. According to a 1992 study from Northwestern University Medical Center, only 25 to 30 percent of the injected fat remains after one year. Treatment of acne scars yielded the poorest results. Areas of frequent movement, such as the lips, needed more frequent injections as opposed to more stationary areas, like the forehead.

Torn Earlobes

The earlobe is a soft skin structure. There is no cartilage or bone to support it. It is therefore not surprising that many women experience torn earlobes during their lives. Yet most books on cosmetic surgery make no note of this common problem.

Earlobes generally become torn in one of two ways, both having to do with pierced ears. The usual scenario is where the earring is grabbed and yanked downward, causing the earlobe to rip in two. Another is where the weight of earrings gradually enlarges the hole to the point where it is greatly stretched.

> Pierced ears are the main cause of torn earlobes.

In either of these situations, the repair process is the same. Since skin that is intact will not attach to another piece of intact skin, the trick with earlobe repair is to connect raw skin to raw skin. To connect intact skin to intact skin would be like taping your fingers together for a day—as soon as the tape is released, the two intact surfaces are free to separate. But if both fingers had raw surfaces touching each other, then the separation would not take place so easily.

So, in repairing a torn earlobe, both sides are purposely "wounded" to produce a raw surface. This can be accomplished by cutting out a piece of skin on each surface. I have found that wounding the skin with a CO_2 laser can create the needed raw surface.

Some cosmetic surgeons merely stitch the outside skin together while others put in a buried, deep stitch for extra strength. The end result is an earlobe that has been successfully pulled together. Again, the cosmetic surgeon's preference comes into play over whether or not to leave a hole for a post or earring wire. Some prefer to stitch everything completely shut and to put in a new post or wire to the side of the scar two months later. Others leave a small opening at the top of the earlobe sutures, which can be used immediately after the operation.

It takes six to eight weeks for the scar to obtain its maximum strength. This is not invisible mending! There *will* be a visible line at the site of tearing regardless which technique is used.

Questions and Answers

Q. *Is there a hereditary disposition towards developing torn earlobes?*
A. None that has ever been documented. Enough trauma to anyone's earlobe can split it, regardless of hereditary factors.

Q. *Can keloids develop when the earlobe is put back together?*
A. It's highly unlikely. I've never seen it happen and probably with good reason. If the trauma of splitting the earlobe was not enough to cause a keloid, then the process of repairing it is not likely to cause a keloid either.

Q. *Can the earlobes tear again once they are repaired?*
A. If enough trauma is repeated, then a tear can occur again. I advise women not to use heavy earrings in order to avoid a repeat episode. Most are happy to comply. If there is a strong desire to wear heavily weighted earrings, it can be done if the hole is not directly on top of the suture line.

Q. *What do you do if the earlobe tears again?*
A. It can be repaired again. But the scar tissue that is generated makes each repair more difficult.

General Questions about Cosmetic Problems and Treatment

Q. *Are blondes more susceptible to developing wrinkles?*
A. Yes. The lack of skin pigment leaves the underlying collagen more susceptible to the sun's damaging rays.

Q. *How much does a chemical peel hurt?*
A. It depends on the depth of the peel. Lighter peels, like glycolic acid, may sting a lot or not at all. Moderate peels, like those involving trichloracetic acid (TCA), usually do sting. The deeper peels, such as the phenol peels, are quite painful and

may require intravenous sedation during the procedure. Before it, you are sometimes given, for example, acetaminophen (Tylenol) with codeine. For glycolic acid peels, I never premedicate; sometimes I do for TCA peels, depending on the person's reaction to the test site; but I always premedicate when I use phenol.

Q. *Do most physicians do a test site before doing a full face peel?*

A. Many do. Some do not. I think that doing a test site before any peel is a good idea. It lets you know what you can expect in the way of pain, recovery time, and results.

Q. *How long does a chemical peel take to do?*

A. Spot peels may take ten minutes. Full face TCA peels can take up to an hour, especially with taping. Phenol peels are usually done in stages so as to inhibit rapid absorption of the phenol. This means doing one area on one side of the face, waiting a half hour, doing another area, waiting, and so on, until it is completed. The entire process can take two to three hours.

Q. *Could I drive myself home after the peel is completed?*

A. You could after a glycolic acid or TCA peel but not after a phenol peel. Also, if the premedication makes you drowsy, then the answer would be no for a TCA peel as well.

Q. *How much does it hurt when the tape is removed in the twenty-four- to forty-eight-hour period after the peel is put on?*

A. Usually not very much at all. At this stage the skin is oozing somewhat, so that often the tape will just float off.

Q. *How long is the recovery period?*

A. It depends on the depth of the peel. The deeper the peel, the longer the recovery. A glycolic acid peel may look totally fresh within one or two hours, whereas a phenol peel may leave the face pink for six weeks.

Q. *Can I use Retin-A or the AHAs after a chemical peel?*

A. Certainly. Once the skin heals, it is actually helpful to use these agents to maintain skin tone.

Q. *I heard that you can't go into the sun after a peel. Is that true?*

A. You should not go into the sun while the skin is in the healing stage. This again depends on the depth of the peel and the recovery time.

Q. *Earlier you mentioned a minipeel for wrinkles. Is there such a thing as a "mini face lift"?*

A. You can have a brow lift that affects only the forehead, but other than that, a face lift is a face lift and it cannot be done halfway.

Q. *I've heard of people developing numbness on their cheeks after a face lift. How long does that last?*

A. It can last for a short period of weeks or it can last forever. It depends whether the affected nerves can hook up again with neighboring nerves. This, by the way, is a very uncommon complication.

Q. *Doesn't it get hot underneath all of the wrappings?*

A. You bet it does. But it is not intolerable. Instead I would describe it as uncomfortable.

Q. *What do you do if a blood clot forms?*

A. Blood clots can often be removed by the physician simply by nicking the skin and letting out the clot. At other times, a deeper incision may be needed to remove the clot. Sometimes the clot will dissolve and go away by itself.

Q. *I've heard of a technique called the punch-graft dermabrasion. What is that all about?*

A. It is where the pitted scars are removed by "punching" holes in the skin and replacing the holes with plugs of skin that are grafted from another site. When the plugs are firmly in place after several weeks, the entire area is dermabraded. The premise is that the dermabraded plugs will leave a neater scar than a pit that was dermabraded without any plugging.

Q. *Can you have a dermabrasion after a face lift?*

A. Yes. A face lift will get rid of many wrinkles but does nothing for skin coloration, blemishes, and acne scarring. Dermabrasion can correct all of these even after a face lift.

Q. *Do facials and mud packs help get rid of scars from acne?*

A. No. They don't help scarring, but certain techniques can be helpful in the treatment of active acne, which then would prevent scarring. These include incision and drainage of plugged up pores and pustules, liquid nitrogen peeling, or a mild ultraviolet treatment.

Q. *Is it true that popping your own pimples leads to acne scarring?*

A. If an acne lesion is overmanipulated, it could lead to scarring. However, methods such as acne surgery (surgically opening up whiteheads and blackheads) and light peels, done under a physician's supervision, are quite helpful and don't leave scars.

Q. *Is the amount of acne scarring proportional to the number of years you have acne?*

A. Not directly. It is more proportional to the severity of the acne. However, many years of repeated, but less severe, bouts of acne can lead to scarring.

Q. *Will the skin be free of all scarring if a dermabrasion is done correctly?*

A. There will always be some degree of scarring, even with the best of dermabrasions. But there should be marked improvement in comparison to what the skin looked like before.

Q. *Does a dermabrasion hurt more than a chemical peel?*

A. No. Remember that the skin is frozen first before it is dermabraded so that there is no sensation when the dermabrasion is taking place. Premedication should help with any postdermabrasion pain.

Q. *How long does it take for a dermabrasion?*

A. About forty-five minutes to one hour.

Q. *Is the recovery period the same as for a chemical peel?*

A. It depends which type of chemical peel. Dermabrasion recovery is most similar to deep TCA or light phenol peels.

Q. *Does the city where you live influence whether you get wrinkles?*

A. The more sun exposure, the greater the tendency towards wrinkle formation. Higher altitudes, like Denver, may also have a more intense sunlight.

Q. *I've heard that some doctors give two test doses of collagen. Why?*

A. Because even after a negative skin test, there is a very small percentage of people who will still have an allergic reaction.

Those physicians who do two skin tests are trying to eliminate this small but bothersome complication.

Q. *Do some people need more than 1 cc of collagen for their wrinkles?*

A. Yes. Some people may need 2 cc or even 3 cc depending upon what they need to have treated.

Q. *What is the truth about silicone injections?*

A. Despite the bad press that silicone has gotten recently, there are still some physicians who use it. They point to the positive side of silicone, namely its longevity and good cosmetic results. Yet nagging doubts persist regarding silicone's side effects, and it is not FDA approved for injection. Silicone is not anything new to cosmetic surgeons. Its usage has been discussed—both pros and cons—in great detail at medical meetings and in medical journals.

Q. *Can collagen cause reactions, like silicone?*

A. Collagen is a totally different substance than silicone. It is derived from a living substance—bovine collagen—whereas silicone is synthetic. There have been reports of both substances provoking collagen vascular diseases, such as lupus or scleroderma, but that relationship has been strongly questioned by the medical community.

Chapter 7

The Hair and Nails: Care, Cosmetics, and Disorders

Hair problems and, even more so, nail problems are quite difficult to treat, yet they happen to be one of my favorite areas of dermatology to treat. Why? Because so often people have given up hope or have been told by other doctors that nothing can be done.

I'm not saying that I have all the answers. But by combining some basic knowledge, newer treatments, and a little patience, you can get help for some disorders that you might have been resigned to live with.

But first I want to talk about the routine care of your hair and nails. After that I will discuss hair and nail cosmetics, describing them and what to look out for in terms of adverse reactions. I hope some of this information may help you prevent problems down the road.

Hair Care

Shampoos

Shampoos are basically hair cleaners. They are detergents that remove dirt, sweat, oil, and other unwanted elements from the hair. Since detergents alone are very harsh, other ingredients are added, such as softeners, thickeners, fragrance, and preservatives.

Medicated shampoos contain a wide array of ingredients—so much so that reading their labels can be quite an adventure. However, their most important ingredients are zinc pyrithione, sulfur, and tar. The former two have an antibacterial effect, whereas tar acts as an anti-inflammatory agent. The exact mechanism of how these dandruff shampoos work has not been scientifically established, but it is suspected that they reduce inflammation and/or colonies of microorganisms in the scalp. Most recently, a prescription strength shampoo containing the antifungal drug ketoconazole has become available. This drug is used on the assumption that a microscopic degree of scalp fungus that may be present in some people's scalps could contribute to dandruff. However, this theory is far from receiving universal consensus among dermatologists.

> **Dandruff shampoos reduce inflammation and/or colonies of microorganisms in the scalp.**

Many physicians recommend rotating medicated shampoos so that whichever microorganisms are present on your scalp and causing dandruff, they do not become immune to a particular medicated ingredient.

Even in nonmedicated shampoos, the list of ingredients can be long and baffling. The following are some of the most common ones, all of which are detergents: lauryl sulfates, laureth sulfates, sarcosines, sulfosuccinate, sorbitan laurate lauramide diethanolamide, cocamidopropyl betaine, and sodiumlauraminopropionate. The last two ingredients are mild detergents and do not irritate the eyes. They are the ones used in baby shampoos.

Other ingredients that do not cleanse the hairs but may affect texture are sometimes added to the detergents in shampoos. Hair softeners and conditioners make the shampoo a more gentle and kinder substance. Foaming agents make for better lather but not necessarily a better shampoo. Thickeners and ingredients called opacifiers give a creamy consistency to the shampoo but offer no desired or beneficial effect to the hair.

Despite the fact that many of the ingredients in shampoos do not achieve their claimed effect, don't assume that you might as well wash your hair with a plain bar of soap. Shampoos are better for cleaning the hair because they bind up magnesium and calcium films that regular soaps would leave behind on the hair. Soap-treated hair can have a dull appearance, so stick with shampoo for a shinier look.

> **Soap can give hair a dull appearance, so stick with shampoo for a shinier look.**

What is the best shampoo for you? Medicated shampoos are best for dandruff. Baby shampoos work well in kids (who generally don't produce as much scalp oil as adults) but can be used in adults who want to wash their hair every day.

Know your scalp. Shampoos for regular scalps are geared for use in people with a moderate amount of scalp oil production and coarse hair. Oily hair shampoos have stronger detergents and milder conditioners. They work best in teenagers who tend to have the oiliest scalps. Due to their drying nature, these shampoos are not suited for daily use. People with finer hair or dry hair may choose to use dry hair shampoos, which provide mild cleansing and good conditioning. Shampoos for damaged hair are quite similar to dry hair shampoos. They may contain a pH balanced acid to render them milder for people with so-called split ends or for those who have chemically treated hair (from permanent waves, straighteners, hair color, or bleach).

Most commercially manufactured shampoos are similar to one another. They vary mostly in their additives. Some are enriched with aloe, some with protein, and some have vitamins added. You may have to experiment with several brands to find the right one for you.

An important amendment to all of the above must be made concerning the hair of African Americans. It tends to be much drier than the hair of Whites because scalp oil is not easily conveyed along a very curly hair shaft out to the ends of these hairs. Therefore, less frequent shampooing is in order. Once a week or every other week may suffice.

Adverse Reactions to Shampoos

Most shampoos cause no problems. Some may be too drying and make the scalp itch and start flaking. This reaction is usually due to a detergent in the shampoo, but other compounds found in these products can cause such a reaction as well. Especially strong shampoo detergents can actually lead to hair loss in susceptible individuals, although this is a very rare occurrence. Keep in mind that all shampoos will be more drying to the scalp during cold winter weather and, in general, your scalp reaction will tend to vary with the time of year.

Shampoos will be more drying to the scalp during cold winter weather.

Some individuals have allergic reactions to shampoos. Generally, the preservatives are the culprits. It is common to see these reactions extend beyond the scalp to the ears, forehead, neck, and face. In severe reactions, these areas will be covered with redness, weeping, and crusting.

If you develop anything that you suspect is an allergic reaction on the head and neck area, your shampoo should certainly be thought of as a possible cause. But, when switching shampoos, check the labels. See if you can identify any ingredient that you know irritates you or causes you to have an allergic reaction. Select a shampoo that seems to be as different as possible from the one you had been using. If you switch a number of times and still have problems, you may need to see your dermatologist to undergo patch testing. (See chapter 8.)

Allergic, general hypersensitivity, and toxic reactions can take strange forms and be a real challenge to track down. Here's an example of a rather unusual case but one that typifies the kind of detective work it can require.

The case is one I reported in the *Journal of the American Medical Association* (*JAMA*) in 1980. It involved a person who was admitted to a hospital alcohol treatment program. Every patient in the program took a drug called disulfiram (Antabuse), which causes noxious reactions when alcohol is ingested. With this drug, a patient cannot "sneak a drink" when nobody is looking because he or she will suffer the consequences, and it will become obvious. It so happened that every time a certain participant in the program took a shower, he broke out in a rash. No one could figure out why this was happening. I was called in to investigate the cause of the skin rash. In my questioning of the patient, it appeared that every time he used a particular shampoo, the generalized rash would appear. An examination of the shampoo answered all questions. He was using a shampoo with an added ingredient designed to make the hair appear thicker. The extra ingredient was beer. Apparently, the beer in the shampoo was being absorbed into his system and reacting with the Antabuse he was taking. Thus a little bit of detective work revealed the source of the rash.

Since we can absorb many substances through our skin and into our system, I suspected that although he was not imbibing, his skin was. That, in combination with the disulfiram, was probably the cause of the rash. Confirmation came when he stopped the shampoo and the rash cleared up completely.

Nail Care

People are often not sure of the best way to trim the nails. Nails can be rounded at the tip but should be left square at the corners. This maximizes nail strength and helps avoid ingrown nails. Clippers are better than scissors for squaring the edges. Ingrown toenails are a common menace often precipitated by improper footwear. The constant jamming of the feet into narrow shoes can cause the nail to dig into the flesh. Inflammation, tenderness, and pus formation may accompany ingrown toenails. A simple method of treatment is to place a piece of cotton under the corner of the nail. This lifts up the nail, encourages it to stop pushing into the surrounding skin, and cuts down the chances of inflammation and infection. It also allows the nail to grow in the proper direction. Good nail grooming is more important than any nail cosmetic.

> To avoid ingrown nails, trim them so that they are left square at the corners.

Cosmetics for the Hair and Nails

Although a cosmetic is most often thought of as a product used on the face—like lipstick, foundations, and rouge—any product that people use for the purpose of feeling and being attractive, and improving or beautifying the physical appearance of their skin, hair, and nails can be called a cosmetic. According to the *American Heritage Dictionary*, the word "cosmetic" is defined as "a preparation . . . designed to beautify the body by direct application." This would include hair dyes, permanent waves, hair straighteners, and hair sprays, as well as nail polish, nail hardeners, and the like.

Hair Dyes

Current estimates have it that 40 percent of women and 5 percent of men dye their hair. Permanent hair dyes work by coloring the outer part of the hair shaft. This is accomplished by a process known as oxidation—the combining of oxygen with one or more ingredients of the hair dye. Thus, hair dye products come in two packages, one

> Forty percent of women and five percent of men dye their hair.

containing the active ingredients and the other containing the oxidizer. The most common ingredient in permanent hair dyes is paraphenylenediamine. Although this is the mainstay of hair dyes, the law prohibits its use for hair around the eye, the eyebrows, and the eyelashes. The reason is simple: the risk of allergic or irritant reaction, although small, poses a potential threat to eyesight.

Allergic reactions to paraphenylenediamine range from mild to wild. Estimates are that one out of every one hundred thousand applications of permanent hair dye leads to an allergic reaction. If you develop a reaction to hair dye while using the product, stop right away. Since almost all permanent hair dyes contain that ingredient, if you do have an allergic reaction to such a dye, it may signal an end to the use of this method of coloring. For, even though the hair dye is permanent, it must periodically be reapplied in order to cover that part of the hair shaft (often referred to as "the root") that newly grows out from the scalp.

> One out of every 100,000 applications of permanent hair dye leads to an allergic reaction.

One important fact to bear in mind with paraphenylenediamine allergy is the phenomenon of cross-reactivity. This refers to the capacity to develop an allergy to substances that are similar to something else to which you are already allergic. Cross-reactivity can occur between paraphenylenediamine and PABA, the backbone of many sunscreens. This is not to say that all people who are allergic to the one will be allergic to the other. But those who know that they are sensitive to hair dyes should look for PABA-free sunscreens rather than tempting fate. And if you are allergic to PABA, you should consider avoiding products with paraphenylenediamine.

> Those who are sensitive to hair dyes should look for PABA-free sunscreens.

Unfortunately, sensitization to a topically applied cosmetic product can also involve cross-reactivity to medications. In the case of paraphenylenediamine these include topical or injectable anesthetics containing benzocaine or procaine. Procaine is also an ingredient in certain heart medications. An oral medication group, the sulfonamides, can also cross-react with paraphenylenediamine. I think by now you must be getting the picture. Through cross-reactivity, paraphenylenediamine allergy can be associated with allergies to some important medicines.

If you develop an allergy to permanent hair dyes, or if you want to avoid these dyes, a semipermanent hair dye may be used.

These last for six to ten shampoos, and several types are available. They don't require oxidation and therefore operate on a different principle than their permanent counterparts. Unfortunately, about one out of four individuals sensitive to the paraphenylenediamine in the permanent dyes will develop a reaction to semipermanent hair dyes. Thus, if you have been sensitive to permanent dyes or you tend to get allergic reactions, it may be wise to undergo patch testing to the semipermanent dye before using it.

For those who are allergic to both permanent and semipermanent dyes, some other alternatives do exist. Natural hair dyes, derived from plant sources, have been used for centuries. The most famous of these is henna. Although henna does not cause allergic reactions as frequently as permanent hair dyes, on rare occasions it has been known to cause hives. Also, it has been reported that the ammonium persulfate booster used with henna can cause asthma in hairdressers but not in their clients.

Another alternative to permanent hair dyes is the gradual hair dyes. These are derived from metallic salts and, as their name suggests, they gradually color the hair. Unfortunately, they do not impart as natural a look to the hair as other hair dyes do. In addition, the hair becomes more brittle and an odor may persist.

Temporary hair dyes, which last just twenty-four hours, are derived from textile dyes.

Finally, there are temporary hair dyes, which last just twenty-four hours. They are derived from textile dyes, but the necessity for frequent reapplication renders them impractical.

Hair Bleaches

Hair bleaches may present problems of their own. Often, the active ingredient is hydrogen peroxide, but they usually also contain an alkaline mix, which speeds up oxidation. When bleaches are too strong, they can irritate the skin. Hairs may break easily, which can be very distressing. An unusual reaction to hair bleaches is hives—big, itchy, red bumps. These hives, or wheals as they are sometimes called, are caused by the release of a substance called histamine from the mast cells of the skin. They can be present just on the scalp or all over the body. In severe cases, fainting can occur as a result of the generalized release of histamine.

Hair Sprays

Hair sprays are seldom the cause of allergic reactions. When they do affect skin, they produce shampoo-like allergic symptoms on the scalp, the face, and neck.

Permanents

Permanents, also called permanent waves or perms, create curls or waves that are longer lasting than those achieved by setting the hair with curlers or by using various forms of curling and waving irons. The effective ingredient in permanents is an alkaline chemical, alkali-thioglycolate. The lotion that contains it is applied to hair that has been rolled into curls and then subjected to heat or cold. With the perms that use heat, if it is excessive it can singe the hair, causing it to break easily. Even worse, the scalp can be burned deeply, and when that happens irreversible hair loss can result.

With either the hot or the cold method, an irritant reaction from the alkali may produce pimples and blisters in some people. A true allergic reaction is less common than the irritant reaction, but an allergic reaction can occur. If it does, it often takes on the same appearance as the irritant reaction. In either case, redness, itchiness, and scaling can be reactions to permanent waves. If any of these symptoms appear while the wave is being applied, it is wise to stop the process to avoid any further problems.

Hair Straighteners

Hair straighteners are often thought of as involving the same chemicals that permanent wave products do. However, only on rare occasions do hair straighteners use the alkali-thioglycolate mix found in permanent wave solutions, and they are only temporary in their effect. Petrolatum (Vaseline-type) preparations are generally used to straighten the hair, as are waxes, paraffins, and gums.

Hair straighteners are generally safer than permanents.

There are fewer problems with hair straighteners than with permanents because the basic ingredients are more inert and thus less toxic to the skin. However, when an alkali-thioglycolate mix is used in straighteners, it can produce the same reactions that the permanent waves do. Also, when heavy amounts of the petrolatum are used and get on the face, acne can result due to a mechanical plugging up of the pores. All in all, however, hair straighteners are fairly safe products to use.

Nail Polish

Nail polish, also referred to as nail enamel, contains several main ingredients, such as film formers, plasticizers, solvents, and colorants. The film formers provide hardness and adhesion, while the plasticizers impart flexibility. All ingredients are dissolved in a solvent, with colorants and fillers added to obtain the desired appearance.

Nail polish, or enamel, is made out of several chemical ingredients, including solvents, colors, and plasticizers. The component that most commonly causes allergic reactions is the thermoplastic resin, which is used to increase the adherence of the nail polish. The resin also serves to make the nails glossier.

> Nail polish reactions are not as severe as allergies to artificial nails.

Several things must be taken into consideration with regard to allergy to nail polish. First of all, reactions are not as severe as with allergies to artificial nails. Secondly, as the nail polish dries, it has less allergic potential. Finally, the rash produced by nail polish sensitivity is most often not around the nails. More often than not, delicate areas of the body that the nail polish touches are affected. These include the eyelids, the face, and the

> Rashes from nail polish can occur on delicate areas of the body touched by the nails.

genitals. One way around this problem is to use nail enamel without the thermoplastic resin. Several nail polish products of this sort, often referred to as hypoallergenic, are available on the market. However, this type of nail polish is not as elegant in appearance and has more of a tendency to chip and peel.

Nail polish removers contain solvents that dissolve the enamel. Depending upon how strong the solvent is and how sensitive the surrounding skin is, an irritant reaction can occur. Again, this is not anywhere as severe as an allergy to artificial nails.

Nail Hardeners

Nail hardeners act by causing some dehydration. Formerly, formaldehyde was used as their main ingredient, but due to numerous instances of allergic reactions, it has been replaced by more inactive substances, such as acetates, nylon, toluene, and polyamide resins. Hardeners are actually clear nail polish with different con-centrations of solvents and resins.

Nail hardeners contain various ingredients, one of which may be formaldehyde—a preservative found also in clothing, shoes, cosmetics, antiperspirants, and many other products we come in contact with daily. It is a very common source of allergy. Reactions to nail hardeners, however, are usually mild with no potential for any permanent nail damage.

Artificial Nails

There are two kinds of artificial nails—preformed nails and sculp-tured ones. Preformed nails come in a variety of colors, shapes, and sizes. They are glued onto the existing nail and are temporary. The acrylic glue is deliberately weak in order to keep the natural nail from being injured when the preformed nail is taken off.

Sculptured nails offer several advantages but with them come disadvantages. They afford a more natural look and allow for vari-ation in the length of the nail. In fact, the reason they are sculpted is so they can fit onto the ends of the natural (the real) nail. This al-lows the newly constructed nail to be shaped to whatever length desired. Strong acrylics are then applied in order to integrate your own nail with the sculptured one so that the new nail looks natural.

Their drawbacks, however, are several. These included infec-tions from unsterile application, nail splitting as the real nail grows, and thinning of the underlying natural nail. Allergic reactions can also occur, and they can be severe.

Maintenance is a must with sculptured nails. They should be applied on top of a cleaned and disinfected natural nail, and they should also be touched up every two to three weeks. These mainte-nance guidelines are for health as well as cosmetic reasons.

Maintenance is a must with sculptured nails.

Artificial nails are the most common source of nail product problems. The acrylics used with artificial nails are strong sensitiz-ers, and allergic reactions can be the result. As will be demon-strated in the case discussed below, these can be severe. Although most nails grow back normally, prolonged use of these acrylics can damage the nail matrix, which is where the nail is manufactured. That can result in permanent deformity.

Whenever I discuss adverse reactions to nail products I can't help but remember a particular patient who came to see me. Artificial nails had been applied to all of her fingers, and these nails had then been wrapped so that they would adhere better. She felt a stinging sensation after a day or two but was told that she should keep the wrap on so that the nails would stay in place. After forty-eight hours of increasing itching, burning, and pain, she removed the wrap and, much to her dismay, what she saw was a mess. The skin around the nails was red, swollen, and oozing. The worst part was that the artificial nails had indeed hardened onto her own nails and were impossible for her to remove.

After some aggressive topical and oral therapy, she began to improve. However, even for months afterwards, her nails were somewhat deformed. Eventually she made a full recovery from this hypersensitivity reaction. But not everyone is so lucky.

Nail Wraps

Silk or linen wraps may add to the beauty of the nail. An acrylic liquid is applied to the nail followed by the placement of a silk or linen cloth. Then, several more layers of acrylic are applied on top to seal the cloth. Linen wraps are stronger than silk wraps. The wraps can be left on for weeks at a time. Their purpose is cosmetic—they don't contribute to strengthening the nail.

Hair Growth Disorders

Women can suffer from two general types of hair problems—an undesirable decrease in scalp hair and an unwanted abundance of body hair, especially on the face. Both types of problems will be discussed below.

The normal cycle of scalp hair growth and hair loss (see chapters 2) does not involve any substantial hair thinning or baldness. Thus, when thinning or balding does occur in women it is evidence of a problem—and one that causes a great deal of very understandable psychological distress.

In order to treat hair loss, it is important to distinguish among the several different types of hair loss patterns that exist and to first determine if true hair loss is actually taking place.

As discussed in chapter 2, the average scalp loses seventy-five to one hundred hairs a day. That means that those hairs you see at the bottom of the shower do not necessarily indicate an advancing hair loss problem but just normal daily loss.

Alopecia Areata

One type of localized hair loss is called alopecia areata. This involves round bald spots. It can result from stress or illness, but most cases are due to unknown causes. Alopecia areata resembles ringworm but not precisely: alopecia areata is not scaly, and its borders are very sharply defined. Also, alopecia areata will show no microscopic evidence of fungus, whereas ringworm, which *is* a fungal infection, does. Alopecia areata will often go away by itself, although it can get worse. But to say that it goes away only means that new bald spots won't occur, not that hair will necessarily regrow, either at all or satisfactorily, on the site of the bald spots that have already occurred. Treatment must sometimes be employed for the spots that remain. The treatment used is topical or injectable corticosteroids.

Telogen Effluvium

Another common type of hair loss is telogen effluvium (see also chapter 4). Rather than being a localized bald spot, this condition involves generalized scalp hair thinning. As with alopecia areata, it may be precipitated by stress or illness, and it usually also resolves spontaneously. Again, injections of steroids or sometimes hormonal extracts can be helpful.

Androgenetic Alopecia (Female Pattern Thinning)

A hair loss disorder that is quite prevalent is androgenetic alopecia, also known as female pattern thinning. This is a hereditary thinning of the hair at the central part of the scalp. It is caused by androgen hormones. The onset can occur at any age, from the twenties on up. The problem is a lack of replacement of lost hairs. In this condition, women may first notice hair thinning as a widening at the part. However, it is imperative to note that, unlike men with male pattern thinning, women with androgenetic alopecia never go completely bald.

Women with androgenetic alopecia generally have normal menses and normal pregnancies. However, some dermatologists feel that certain blood studies for hormones should be done in younger women with androgenetic alopecia.

I don't know how many women with androgenetic alopecia have said to me, "But no one else in my family has this." While female pattern thinning *is* a genetic trait, it is of polygenic inheritance—meaning there is more than one gene regulator involved. And, when more than one regulator is needed to produce a trait, the chances of that trait's occurring are considerably diminished. Hence, this condition may skip several generations or even be modified by different genetic combinations and influences.

In androgenetic alopecia the hair loss is due to a gradual transformation from a full-sized hair follicle to a dwarfed follicle. Ultimately, even though the hair follicles are all still present, they are miniaturized. This phenomenon is accompanied by hormonal changes taking place within the follicle itself.

On rare occasions, certain hormone abnormalities in women can lead to female pattern thinning. However, these syndromes—unlike androgenetic alopecia—are virilizing syndromes. That is, the hormone abnormalities are often accompanied by masculinizing characteristics, such as a deepening voice, increased facial hair, and irregular menses.

What can be done to prevent or treat androgenetic alopecia? Recently, the popular hair-growing drug minoxidil (Rogaine) has shown promise in halting female pattern thinning. (Although the condition is somewhat hormonally dependent, estrogen replacement therapy used in some menopausal women has not usually shown itself sufficient to protect the hair follicle in the women affected with this condition.)

Rogaine was introduced about ten years ago as an oral antihypertensive. It was discovered that some people taking the drug became hairier. The first studies of its effectiveness for growing hair were performed on men with typical male pattern baldness and thinning. Clinical trials showed that when minoxidil was applied to the scalp, the average number of hairs increased. After thirty-two weeks, 19 percent noticed moderate growth, 40 percent noticed minimal growth, and 41 percent noticed no growth. In those that are helped, it is the vertex (crown) of the scalp that seems to respond the best. Also, the earlier you treat the hair loss, the better the result usually is. This means that men who have been completely bald for years should not expect much in the way of results, whereas men and women who have minimal pattern thinning can count on the best results, especially if the treatment is started early.

The bottom line is this—don't expect dramatic results, but Rogaine can surely help you hold onto what you already have *if* you continue using it. If you stop, you gradually lose those hairs that Rogaine helped to maintain.

Side effects are mild and uncommon. An allergic or irritant rash has been reported in about 7 percent of users. Because its systemic absorption from topical application is minimal there is virtually nothing to worry about in terms of its antihypertensive effect. It is uncommon to see systemic antihypertensive effects like dizziness or lightheadedness.

However, a bothersome side effect that some women complain of is an increase in facial hair. This is presumed to be the result of systemic absorption of the drug through the skin. Systemic absorption, however, isn't always the reason, as is demonstrated in the following case.

A woman patient came to my office complaining of an increase in facial hair while using Rogaine. It turned out that she was applying the medicine to her scalp right before bedtime and some of it was rubbing off on her pillow. As she tossed and turned in her sleep, the residue was rubbed into her face. With the use of a light shower cap to cover the hair and scalp while she slept, no Rogaine rubbed on to her pillow, none got on her face, and the facial hair problem slowly resolved. In that case at least, the facial hair growth was due to inadvertent topical application on the face, not systemic absorption.

There are certain drugs that can enhance Rogaine's performance. Retin-A has been shown to be a very mild hair growth stimulant of its own accord. In addition, Retin-A can prepare the skin so that Rogaine penetrates better.

Estrogen preparations, either applied topically or injected into the scalp, may result in some improvement as well. The hormonal interplay of these different medications is not well known, but there have not been any side effects reported from their combined use.

Trichotillomania

A very common type of balding in women is also one of the most perplexing. It is a disorder known as trichotillomania, or self-induced hair plucking. This is a problem that is almost exclusive to women, often beginning in childhood. What starts off as innocent hair pulling snowballs into a ritual of often frenzied hair uprooting. It can result in broken hairs or total areas of baldness. Unusual streaks or patches may be present. Permanent destruction of hair follicles can occur if this practice continues. Some women eat the plucked hairs. This condition is often accompanied by feelings of shame and helplessness. The patient is often embarrassed and may feel—and actually be—stigmatized socially.

Some estimates have it that up to two million women in this country have suffered at some point in their lives from one degree of trichotillomania or another. Recently it has been identified as a type of obsessive-compulsive disorder, one that is treatable with psychotropic medication and behavior modification.

For many women, the nightmare continues despite treatment. For them, wigs and elaborate hairstyles serve to hide the defects.

Unwanted Hair

The presence of facial and body hair varies from woman to woman. Excess hair in women, sometimes called "hairiness," is known medically as *hirsutism*. It can run in families and also in certain ethnic groups. However, certain women have excess hair in association with abnormalities in the amounts of estrogen, progesterone, and/or testosterone in their system.

Over the years, many different remedies have been used to combat this problem. Some have a temporary effect while others may actually be permanent. The newer techniques include drug therapy. Shaving with a straight blade is one of the ways women remove unwanted hair. However, irritation and nicking are common problems, and not only can these be uncomfortable, when they occur on the face they are unsightly in themselves and can call attention to the fact that the woman has shaved—a fact many women would prefer to keep private. Electric shavers are gentler and therefore better suited for the removal of facial or body hair in women. And, yes, today's electric shavers can shave as close as a blade.

Depilatories are chemicals that remove hairs by dissolving them. Quite a few over-the-counter brands are available. They are commonly used for contouring eyebrows, removing unwanted hair from the face—primarily from the area above the upper lip—and reducing the need for shaving the legs and underarms. Some brands are stronger than others and as such, caution should be used when applying them to the face. The ubiquitous chemical combination of alkali and thioglycolate is found in these products, although in depilatories it is much more concentrated than in permanents or hair straighteners, meaning using these products will not cause hair loss. Although the alkaline nature of the compound gets rid of hairs, it also can irritate the skin. Ditto for the alkali-sulfide combinations, which tend to be stronger than their thioglycolate counterparts and also bring with them that objectionable sulfur smell. Perfumes are sometimes added to mask the odor, but individuals who are sensitive to perfumes may develop allergic reactions. As with shaving, the effects of depilatories are only temporary.

Waxing is another mechanical method for the removal of hair anywhere on the body. An adhesive substance is applied to the skin and then quickly removed. The hair that became embedded in it is pulled out as it is removed. Local irritation may result from this, because this process constitutes a trauma to the skin. This method is reasonably safe, but repeated traumatic elimination of the hair may cause permanent deformity of the follicle, leading to crooked hairs. Also, some of these products contain perfumes and chemicals, which always can produce allergic reactions.

Plucking, whose fancier name is manual epilation, is an effective, temporary means of hair elimination, but it can also disrupt the follicle and produce crooked hairs.

Electrical epilation, more commonly known as electrolysis, aims to permanently remove hair. A very fine needle is attached to an apparatus that generates an electrical current. The needle is inserted down the hair follicle to the base of the hair. The current is then turned on, creating a burst of electricity that, functioning at its best, will permanently destroy the root of the follicle.

The technique does have several drawbacks. First, each one of the electrical shocks is somewhat painful. Multiple attempts may be needed for each follicle in order to destroy it. On occasion, increased pigmentation or even scarring may result—an especially objectionable side effect on the face. And this may last months or may even be permanent in some cases. Depending upon the size of the area being treated, one or two years may be necessary to complete the program.

It should be noted that cosmetics and makeup will adhere better to a woman's face when there is a little bit of "peach fuzz" present. This was brought to light when the American Cancer Society noted that women who had lost their facial hair as a result of chemotherapy found that their makeup did not stick as well as it had before. Apparently, the light hair growth helps to hold facial cosmetics onto the face. Women combating hirsutism should be aware of this fact.

Most recently, advances in pharmacology have enabled physicians to use oral medications in the treatment of hirsutism. As with many medical discoveries, the ability to treat excess hair in women was stumbled upon by accident. A woman who was taking a drug for high blood pressure noticed that her problem with hirsutism was decreasing. The drug she was taking was spironolactone.

Studies done on the effect of this drug on body hair showed that it caused decreased coarseness and decreased darkening of the hair in hirsute women. And the existing body hair was made finer and softer. Using scientific methods, it was determined that the diameter of the hair shaft was smaller and the density of hair growth per square inch was decreased. While hair growth on the face and body diminished, scalp hair was unaffected. That was critical!

Spironolactone acts by blocking certain hormones, so it is not surprising that it has its own share of side effects. Menstrual irregularities and a lowering of blood pressure are the two most common ones. However, these adverse effects usually are not sufficiently serious to cause women to halt treatment when using it for hirsutism.

Investigators have also tried combining spironolactone with other medications, such as the active ingredients in birth control pills or cortisone. The preliminary studies show that the combination therapy may work even better than just spironolactone alone. These early results are still being subjected to more research.

Another medication, called ketoconazole, had a similar route to discovery. It was used successfully for treatment of fungus infections for several years before it was noticed that it blocked the production of a number of hormones, such as testosterone. This led to the use of ketoconazole in conditions such as prostate cancer and precocious puberty. When used in hirsute women, ketoconazole was indeed noted to decrease body and facial hair growth. These beneficial effects occurred only after the patient was on the drug for at least six months. Potential side effects, however, include liver problems, dryness of the skin, and decreased libido.

As the field of medicine advances towards the twenty-first century, our understanding of the mechanisms of hair growth and hair loss will be expanded. Newer drugs are being developed that have a more specific effect on the hair follicle, and although our current therapies are not perfect they show evidence of hope for the future.

Disorders of the Nails

It is helpful to remember that nails are not there just for appearance and to be groomed but to serve as a protective shield to the fingers and toes. They also make it possible to scratch, to scrape, and to pick things up, especially small objects.

Thus nail problems are more than just unsightly, they can be a real inconvenience and very uncomfortable. Hangnails are often painful and, as most women know, annoying stocking rippers. Thickened toenails cause uncomfortable pressure.

Treating nail disorders is perhaps the most difficult area in the field of dermatology because treatments are often prolonged and not always successful. Part of the problem lies with the nature of nail growth. But, because nail growth is slow, nails are slow to respond to any therapy. However, newer creams, pills, and lasers are now allowing for more successes in treating these disorders.

Distortions of the nail are referred to as nail dystrophies in medical terminology. Several types of dystrophies exist. Some examples are split nails, brittle nails, and thickened nails. These may arise because of the existence of eczema or infections. Or, external factors like nail polish or environmental chemicals can play a causal role. So too can internal disorders like diseases of the thyroid. Mostly, however, nail dystrophies occur simply because the nail becomes weak or defective without any known precipitating factors.

Split Nails

Look closely at those split nails. You might be missing something if you don't. A woman once mentioned to me in passing that she wished I could do something for her ring fingernail, which was always splitting at the edge. When I examined her nail I noticed a slight redness under the area where the nail was splitting. Trimming back the nail revealed a small red bump growing out of the nail bed. A biopsy revealed a glomus tumor—an uncommon nail bed growth—that had split the overlying nail in two. Upon removal of the glomus tumor, the new nail that grew back was perfectly normal.

Brittle Nails

When evaluating brittle nails, you must consider what might have precipitated the problem. Repetitive hand washing causes a wet/dry cycle that tends to dry out the nails. Use of harsh detergents or chemicals is another factor. Identifying and eliminating these triggers are essential to treatment.

The use of moisturizers to rehydrate brittle nails is the mainstay of its therapy. There is a bit of controversy regarding the use of nail polish with brittle nails. Some experts feel that nail polish is beneficial because it slows the evaporation of water from the nail plate, while others feel that the ingredients in nail polish are too drying to the already brittle nail. You really have to see what works best with your nails if you have this problem.

Thickened Nails

An exaggerated form of toenail thickening known as *onychogryphosis* is common in older people. The toenails can become tough and markedly thickened and actually curve to the side, often digging into the adjacent toe. Frequent clippings, laser debulking, or nail removal is often helpful.

For regular thickened nails, known as *onychauxis,* similar treatments are employed. Either concentrated urea or acid—both of which soften the nail—is used. The CO_2 laser can be used to slowly burn off the thickened layers of the nail. I have found that when done properly this should be a painless procedure. Surgical removal of the nail, after local anesthesia, is another option. Usually, although not always, a new, healthy nail grows back.

Nail Infections

By now you probably have noticed that practically all of the medical terms for nail problems have the root *onych* in them. It's the Latin and Greek term for *nails* (as well as *claws*). *Mycosis* refers to disease caused by a fungus. Hence, *onychomycosis* is the name given to fungal infection of the nails, popularly referred to as "fungus nails." It is the most common of the nail infections. Toenails are affected more often than fingernails. Infection occurs either from contact with other areas of your body that are infected or from contact with a fungal infection on another person or from a fungus-infected area, like the floor of a shower. When this condition affects the nails they become yellowish, crumbly, and thickened.

Sometimes, the only symptom of onychomycosis is a superficial white patch. Thus it can be easily missed, and the fungus then would spread. The white patch is usually crumbly rather than smooth. So, pay attention to white patches on the nails.

If the affected portion of the nail is small, it can be cut away or lasered off. If the area is larger or if many nails are affected, several options exist. The offending nails may be removed, although this does require local anesthesia. Often, the treatment of choice is oral antifungal medications. Concentrated urea or acid pastes may also be used on the nails directly. These slowly eat away at the nails and the fungus they contain. Then, newer, healthy nails grow in. Combinations of all of the above methods may also be used. These treatments may take up to a year to work, because the infected nails are only slowly replaced with a healthy nail since, as stated earlier, nails grow so slowly.

A method that I have found particularly helpful for ingrown nails is the partial matrixectomy. This is where the offending portion of the nail—usually about one sixth of the total nail—is removed. Its root is also destroyed, with the result that *no* nail regrowth occurs at that site. The CO_2 laser is an effective tool for this and is associated with very little postoperative pain (as opposed to other techniques, which are associated with more postoperative discomfort).

Nail Psoriasis

Psoriasis (see chapter 8) can attack the nails in addition to the skin. Psoriatic nails can have pits, splits, or a very characteristic "oil-drop sign." This is a yellowish discoloration that is broadly distributed throughout the nails. Psoriatic nails may benefit from oral or topical PUVA (*p*soralen plus *u*ltra*v*iolet *A*) treatments—a type of ultraviolet therapy. Other treatment methods, such as creams, ointments, and even injections into the nail root, have been tried for this condition, all having some success.

Nail Signs of Internal Disorders

Nail problems may be a clue, sometimes the first clue, to an internal disorder.

Clubbing of the nails—a change in the angle of the nails—is commonly found in people with lung disease. Normally, when you look at the nail sideways, it is angled slightly upwards from the skin level. In clubbing, there is a complete loss of this angle, and the nail is flattened and somewhat broader. Just why the nail changes direction in response to lung disease is unknown. But the condition is well known as being a sign of emphysema and lung cancer.

In people with low thyroid problems (hypothyroidism), the nails get softer and the skin gets doughy and thick.

Nail Reactions and Injuries from Occupational Exposures

The nail is also a frequent victim of occupational exposures. Chemicals, trauma, allergies, and radiation can all produce work-related nail problems. Those whose work exposes their hands to water a great deal can develop *paronychia.* This is an inflammation of the skin surrounding the nail, often caused by yeast infections. Chronic paronychia can lead to permanent disfigurement of nails. Treatment is with antibiotics and avoiding exposing the hands to water.

Nail injuries are common among athletes. The nail may be broken or pitted. Trauma may cause a painful accumulation of blood—a hematoma—underneath the nail. Getting the trapped blood out relieves the pressure and pain. Interestingly, the frequent use of aspirin or nonsteroidal anti-inflammatory drugs, like Motrin and Advil, increases the likelihood of hematoma formation. That's because many of these drugs tend to thin out the blood.

Workers in beauty salons are also at risk for developing nail problems. Hairdressers may develop *onycholysis,* or nail splitting, as a result of hair fragments being trapped under the nail. This can lead to infection or allergy. Constant handling of hair dye may stain the nails. Exposure to nail acrylics can cause allergic reactions, some of which are severe.

Typing may cause the nails to split or chip. Constant trauma may bring on or aggravate a case of psoriasis of the nails. Dentists and dental hygienists may either suffer from paronychia, nail trauma, or radiation damage if their nails are exposed to x-rays. This can occur from holding the films in their patients' mouths. Fortunately, this practice is on the wane, as most x-rays are now held in the mouth with mechanical devices.

Half-and-Half Nails

Nails that are called half-and-half nails are a sign of kidney disease. Their name is taken from the fact that the lower white part of the nail extends about halfway up the nail instead of occupying just a very small part of the bottom of the nail. Again, what causes this is not well understood.

Terry's Nails

Another nail disorder, *Terry's nails,* is similar to half-and-half nails, but appears in people who have cirrhosis of the liver. Here the whiteness extends all the way to the tip of the nail, leaving just a small, pink band at the edge. The cause for this is felt to be a lack of albumin. Improvement in the liver disease is accompanied by a resolution of the nail problems.

Nail Transplants

One interesting surgical note is worth mentioning. You've heard of heart transplants and kidney transplants. How about nail transplants? There is such a thing! Recent surgical journals describe transplanting a person's own toenail to their thumbnail area. In the process it is not enough to transplant the nail. The nail root (matrix) must be transplanted with it to ensure continued growth of the nail. These autologous (from the person's own body) nail transplants are helpful for people without fingernails, who have difficulty picking things up.

Chapter 8

Other Skin Conditions, Diseases, and Reactions

During the course of this book I've described many skin conditions, diseases, and reactions. Some I could only mention in passing. Others weren't discussed at all but deserve attention because so many women experience them sometime in their lives. Hence this chapter.

First is a discussion of allergic and irritant skin reactions, including occupational skin disorders. Next, I talk about the well-known diseases and conditions that affect the skin, like skin cancer. The chapter closes with a discussion of skin diseases and conditions that, although they cause considerable suffering, are less well known and tend to occur with less frequency.

But do remember, if you are looking for information about a skin disease or condition and you don't find it here, check the index at the back of the book, for it may have been discussed earlier in the book. This is not to say that you will find mention of *every* possible skin problem between the two covers of this book. That would be too much to ask even for a huge medical text devoted only to dermatological diseases.

My hope is that this material may help you prevent problems and better understand any skin conditions you might already have.

Allergic and Irritant Reactions

An adverse skin reaction can occur in response to virtually any substance, although some things are more likely than others to cause such reactions. The skin signs of these reactions generally are rashes, blisters, or hives and can result from topical, ingested, or inhaled exposure. With topical exposure, the source is often something that has been applied to the skin, as with a shampoo or perfume, or a plant. However, ingested substances, like food and medicine, sometimes are the culprit. Dry products, which are fine enough to be airborne and inhaled, or chemicals and paints, whose droplets can be carried in the air, can also cause skin problems.

But, regardless what triggers the skin reaction, there are basically two types: (1) allergic and (2) irritant. I will first discuss their differences and then the features they share.

Allergic Skin Reactions

Allergic reactions can be thought of as a kind of protective mechanism gone haywire. The immune system is in the business of protecting the body against substances that the body comes in contact with that could be harmful to it. Occasionally, however, it puts up a misguided fight. The immune system's protective response turns into an overreaction. The histamine that is released from the mast cells in the blood and tissues causes many of the familiar signs and symptoms of allergy (and sometimes odd and unfamiliar ones, too). The substance that triggered the immune system to react this way is called an *allergen.*

Anything can act as an allergen. Why certain things do, why they do at certain times and not at others (allergies sometimes come and go), and why some things act as allergens to some people and not to others are all questions for which there are still no fully satisfactory answers. But it *is* known that certain substances (foods, medicines, or other chemicals) tend to trigger allergic reactions more often than others do—like peanuts and poison ivy. And, it is also known that in order to have a true allergic reaction to anything, you must have already had at least one previous exposure to it or to a substance that bears considerable similarity to it chemically (see discussion of cross-reactivity in chapter 5).

It is also important to realize that you can become allergic to things even if you have been exposed to them for many years without problems. The reason for this is also unknown, but something apparently triggers the immune system to perceive the formerly tolerated substances as an allergen and thus an enemy.

> **You can become allergic to things even if you have been exposed to them for many years without problems.**

Skin allergies usually persist for many years, although after age seventy, when the immune system tones down, allergies become less frequent. Allergic skin reactions take on different forms—they can be itchy, red rashes, or blisters, or, occasionally, hives, sometimes called wheals.

Common sources of skin allergy at home and on the job include rubber, fabric, and dyes. Skin reactions to earrings, the metal

> **Allergic skin reactions take on different forms—itchy, red rashes, blisters, or hives.**

back of a watch, belt buckles, and bra hooks can be traced to their nickel content. Allergies to dyes or colors in clothing or shoes may cause your skin to break out. Rubber is another frequent culprit. The thin latex (rubber) disposable gloves that are used in the "universal precautions" against infection are an occasional cause of skin reactions for women and men in medicine, nursing, and dentistry. And, women who are allergic to rubber sometimes have problems in beauty salons. The rubber headrest attached to the shampoo tray can be a source of sensitivity. Allergies to rubber can mean problems for women (and men) who use latex condoms for birth control and disease prevention.

Urticaria, or hives, that is, itchy, red bumps, can result from inhaling things to which you may be allergic. Grasses and trees are some of the usual culprits. Sophisticated allergy tests have been devised to test for allergies of this nature.

Irritant Reactions

Irritant reactions differ from allergies in that no prior exposure is necessary. Irritants can be caustic substances—such as acids or alkalis— or milder chemicals—such as solvents or detergents. These are frequently found in household cleansers and

> **Irritant reactions differ from allergies in that no prior exposure is necessary.**

many products used by chemists, carpenters, secretaries, doctors, artists, and people in many other occupations.

Similarities between Allergic and Irritant Reactions

Irritant and allergic skin reactions look very much alike, and both can set the stage for further problems. For, skin that is dry, cracked, reddened, or raw—no matter what the cause—is more easily irritated by other chemicals and can be have an increased susceptibility to allergic reactions. In addition, such skin provides an easy breeding ground for infection.

There is one kind of skin reaction—called a *photosensitive reaction*—that can be either allergic or irritant in nature. What happens is that the skin reacts to a combination of a particular substance *and* sunlight. The irritant variety is referred to as a *phototoxic reaction.* These reactions usually look like sunburn. *Photoallergic reactions* tend to be itchy and scaly.

Photosensitive reactions can be triggered by natural sunlight or even sunlight that passes through window glass. The light that passes through glass is the UVA spectrum, and it is the UVA (as opposed to UVB) rays that can set off the reaction.

Making the Diagnosis

The standard way of determining whether an irritant or allergic reaction has occurred is via a patch test. The substance one wants to test is applied to a patch. This is then placed on an area of clear, clean skin to see if a reaction takes place. If you are indeed allergic to the substance, a noticeable rash will be detected within twenty-four to seventy-two hours after the patch was applied. Sometimes several patch tests are done at one time, each testing a different substance.

In the case of testing for photosensitive reactions, the applied substance must be exposed to ultraviolet light. It is then checked two to three days later.

As with other medical tests, patch test results can occasionally be false positives or false negatives, leading the physician astray in getting to the root of the problem. Unfortunately, and to the frustration of many patients and doctors, the process of finding the specific cause of a reaction is an inexact science. It often requires close observation by patient and doctor as well as trial and error in eliminating suspects, just as with all good detective work.

Skin Reactivity in Women

Medical science has recently documented something that women have probably known intuitively for years—the skin is more sensitive just before the menstrual period. In 1988, a British study demonstrated that some women had positive patch tests to certain substances before their period but negative results to patch tests of those same substances ten days later. All of this points towards a premenstrual cutaneous hypersensitivity—a sort of premenstrual syndrome (PMS) of the skin!

Occupational Skin Disorders

Skin problems can result from certain occupational or lifestyle practices. In fact, these are one of the leading causes of disability in the United States. Hand dermatitis from frequent water exposure affects bartenders, waitresses, nurses, doctors, janitorial workers, housewives, artists, and artisans; in other words, anyone whose work involves a lot of hand exposure to water and/ or chemicals. The constant wet/dry cycle dries

> **Skin problems from work and lifestyle practices are a leading cause of disability in the United States.**

out the skin on the hands, rendering it red, cracked, and bleeding. Once that occurs, the skin becomes even more sensitive to water and solvents. So it is a vicious circle.

Treatment ideally should involve avoiding water or chemical exposure as much as possible. But, few of us can or are willing to make the kind of changes in our work that such avoidance would require. So the next best thing is to use rubber gloves (or plastic ones, if you are sensitive to latex). And, whenever the hands do get wet, a liberal amount of moisturizer should be applied and rubbed in. Topical corticosteroid creams are useful as well. Avoidance of detergents, chemicals, and soaps will allow the skin to heal to its normal state. (See chapter 7 for a discussion of nail reactions and injuries that result from occupational exposures and work-related tasks.)

Foot Problems

> **Feet enclosed in hot, sweaty shoes all day long are the perfect breeding ground for fungus infections.**

Sometimes jobs require you to stand a lot or wear high-heeled shoes. And you rarely get a chance to change your shoes while at work. Having your feet enclosed in hot, sweaty shoes all day long provides the perfect breeding ground for fungus infections. Fungus between the toes can turn the skin red or white and make it moist, scaly, or itchy. Fungus on the soles typically makes the skin scaly and itchy. Popularly known as 'athlete's foot,' its treatment involves not only topical antifungal agents but also good aeration of the feet to eliminate the breeding ground for fungus. High-heeled shoes can cause skin problems. Pressure on the balls of the feet can lead to the formation of calluses. Squeezing toes into small spaces precipitates ingrown toenails. Friction on the sides of toes can cause an irritant dermatitis and/or callus formation.

> High-heeled shoes can cause skin problems like calluses, ingrown toenails, and irritant dermatitis.

Well-Known Diseases and Conditions That Affect the Skin

The Collagen Vascular Diseases

As the name implies, collagen vascular diseases affect the collagen and vascular (blood vessel) components of the skin and many of the internal organs as well. The effects on the skin are confined primarily to the dermis—the layer right beneath the epidermis (see chapter 2).

Lupus

While lupus is a collagen vascular disease it is also a member of another class of diseases—the autoimmune diseases, called that because the body's immune system turns against itself. Lupus affects women primarily—about one out of every thousand. It can be very mild with only occasional skin involvement or it can involve many body organs and be fatal.

The two types of lupus that affect the skin only are *discoid lupus* and *subacute cutaneous lupus*. In both, a red, scaly rash appears on the skin, especially in sun-exposed areas. On the face the rash affects the cheeks and runs across the bridge of the nose. It looks something like a red butterfly and, as a result, it has come to be referred to as a "butterfly rash." Repeated episodes of the rash, or flare-ups, can lead to scarring. When this occurs on the patient's face, it is, quite understandably, very troubling.

> In lupus, a rash that affects the cheeks and the bridge of the nose is called a "butterfly rash."

About 10 percent of those who have the skin-only types of lupus will, unfortunately, go on to develop systemic lupus. Systemic lupus—its complete name being *systemic lupus erythematosus,* or "SLE"—most commonly involves the kidneys, lungs, joints, and the skin. In fact, almost any part of the body can be affected. Indeed, the heart, nervous system, eyes, liver, and the gastrointestinal tract can also suffer the effects of this disease. Treatment for all types of lupus is with corticosteroids and/or other medications.

As is the case with so many diseases, the path to discovering that someone has lupus often varies considerably from patient to patient. I recall the time that I saw an executive, a woman in her late twenties, who felt overworked. She enjoyed her job, but she was fatigued and sometimes achy after a long day at the office. To get away from it all, she took a week's vacation in Mexico. I saw her at the end of her vacation because she had what she felt was unusual for her—a sunburn. This woman had never burned before despite numerous trips to sunny climates.

As it turned out, she was very right to be concerned. This was no ordinary sunburn. It involved the bridge of the nose and the upper cheeks but spared the rest of her face. I ran a simple blood count. It revealed a profound anemia. That explained her fatigue problems. Her aches and pains were the beginning of arthritis. Putting the clinical picture together—her symptoms, the form the sunburn took on her face, and the laboratory test results—I was able to pin down the diagnosis. It was systemic lupus erythematosus. Further tests confirmed my suspicions.

Dermatomyositis

Dermatomyositis is another collagen vascular disease—albeit less common than lupus—that has female predominance, just as lupus does. It affects both the skin and the muscles. The skin symptoms can either be very subtle or quite striking. The most characteristic skin sign of dermatomyositis is a purple rash surrounding the eyes— called a "heliotrope rash." When prominent, this can resemble the shape of the markings on the face of a raccoon. Sometimes, in fact, the rash is referred to not as a heliotrope rash but as a "raccoon rash." Purple patches can also appear elsewhere on the face, on the neck, and on the hands. Reddish bumps on the joints, called Gottron's papules, can occur. The muscles become increasingly weak and sore, with the

> The most characteristic skin sign of dermatomyositis is a purple rash surrounding the eyes— called a "heliotrope rash."

shoulder and hip muscles being the most commonly affected. Dermatomyositis has periods of improvement and worsening, but it tends to get progressively worse.

Treatment is similar to that of lupus, with moderate to high doses of steroids often being required. Control, and sometimes cure, can be obtained with the proper medications.

Scleroderma

Scleroderma, like lupus and dermatomyositis, has a higher female than male incidence. The word "scleroderma" means "tight skin." In this disease, the skin around the mouth can become so tightly bound that chewing is made difficult. This same tightening effect on the skin causes a loss of facial lines, making the face expressionless. The symptoms of this condition usually first appear on the hands and the fingers. The skin becomes thick, making simple movements such as bending fingers a chore. Like lupus, scleroderma can involve the kidneys and lungs. Interestingly, there has been some recent evidence linking breast cancer to scleroderma in women. At present the connection is just statistical—a cause and effect relationship has not been established. Scleroderma is progressive and, at present, there is no cure.

The Skin Cancers

Skin cancers are not limited to women, and their increasing incidence is of concern to both sexes. An outdoor lifestyle and a diminishing ozone layer contribute to their development, since sun exposure is the precipitating factor. Use of sunscreen and protective clothing really does decrease the incidence of skin cancer and the precancerous skin problems discussed earlier in the book. As you might suspect, there is a higher rate of skin cancer in fair-skinned people and also in those whose work or lifestyle keeps them outdoors on a daily basis. And, yes, statistics have shown that those bad sunburns you used to get at the beach can predispose you to developing skin cancer at those places on your skin that were burned.

> If you see something on the skin that is growing and becoming irregular in shape, have a dermatologist check it out.

Even though different types of skin cancers have different characteristics, a general rule of thumb is that if a sore doesn't heal or if you see something on the skin that is growing and becoming irregular in shape, it's time to have a dermatologist check it out.

Basal Cell Carcinoma

The most common type of skin cancer—basal cell carcinoma—arises from the basal cell layer of the skin (see chapter 2). Fortunately, it is not an aggressive cancer, but it can erode into the underlying cartilage or bone if left untreated. This form of carcinoma is the most common in the United States. Former President Reagan developed one on his nose, no doubt as a result of his prolonged sun exposure during his Death Valley Days. Former First Lady Barbara Bush had one on her upper lip.

Although basal cell carcinomas are usually smooth and glistening, they can break down and ulcerate. But they never spread to other parts of the body. That is not to say that they can't do plenty of damage. People whose basal cell carcinomas have gone unattended have been known to lose their nose, ears, and even eyes. Certain types of basal cell carcinomas are quite nefarious. These are the sclerosing type, which tend to burrow into the skin and spread sideways.

Basal cell carcinomas appear with increasing frequency from the age of forty on. Treatment is the same as for squamous cell carcinoma (see below).

Squamous Cell Carcinoma

The squamous cell layer of the skin (see chapter 2) can give rise to the deadly squamous cell carcinoma, an aggressive type of skin cancer. It has the appearance of a raised crust that adheres to a reddish base at the sites on the skin that were exposed to the sun. The larger this growth is, the more advanced it tends to be.

As noted above, treatment for both basal cell and squamous cell carcinoma are similar. A number of different methods can be employed. A hard liquid nitrogen freeze often does the trick, but some clinicians feel that this does not offer as high a cure rate as other methods do. Desiccation and curettage is another treatment that is used. This treatment may take two weeks to heal and always leaves a scar of some sort. Lasers, as you might suspect, can also be used, as can simple excisions.

A method of removal that is reserved for only the most resistant cancers is called Mohs' chemosurgery, also known as Mohs' micrographic surgery. Named for Frederick Mohs, M.D., this procedure involves removing the cancer layer by layer and then checking each one microscopically for evidence of residual cancer. When the layer is reached that no longer contains any microscopic evidence of carcinoma, the cancer is deemed to have been fully removed.

Keep in mind that none of these procedures is foolproof. Although cure rates may vary from 95 to 99 percent, both squamous cell and basal cell carcinoma can come back, even with Mohs' chemosurgery. In order to catch a recurrence as early as possible, frequent follow-up visits are so important.

Malignant Melanoma

Malignant melanoma is one of the deadliest of all known cancers, not just skin cancers. It is a black growth on the skin, which usually has an irregular shape. It can arise from a mole that is already present but can also just simply appear. Many different types of malignant melanomas exist. Some are flat and spread sideways, while others are bumpy and spread upwards and downwards. Rarely, a melanoma devoid of pigment—referred to as an *amelanotic melanoma*—will appear. Men and women are affected equally.

> The skin cancer, malignant melanoma, is one of the deadliest of all known cancers.

A melanoma can develop anywhere on the skin, including the palms, the soles, the scalp, and the genitals. The more easily you sunburn, the higher your risk. Both sexes develop it on the areas of skin that tend to be less covered up by clothing and thus more exposed to the sun. Men have a higher percentage of melanomas on the trunk, while women have more of a tendency to form melanomas on the legs. This lends support to those who believe that the sun is the most important factor in the development of this skin cancer. Fair-skinned people have a much higher incidence than darker-skinned people. When Blacks develop melanoma it tends to be on the palms and soles.

Unfortunately, the incidence of malignant melanoma is increasing, doubling every ten years. On the other hand, the cure rate for melanoma is getting better as the years go by, possibly due to earlier detection.

> A melanoma can look very much like an exceedingly common, benign skin growth called a seborrheic keratosis.

Malignant melanoma was mentioned earlier as something that can be confused with seborrheic keratosis (see chapter 3) when making a diagnosis. That a melanoma can look so very much like an exceedingly common, benign skin growth like a seborrheic keratosis suggests that it is always best to let an experienced physician check your skin growths on a regular basis, or when a new growth appears, or when an old growth changes.

Malignant melanomas, due to their grave prognosis, generally warrant an aggressive treatment approach. Almost all melanoma excisions include wide margins around the growth, just to play it safe. The rest of the treatment depends upon the depth of the growth. The original method of determining the depth of the excision was developed by Wallace Clark, M.D., with the different depths being called Clark level I, Clark level II, and so on. A more recent classification system is the simpler Breslow method, which categorizes melanomas as thin (less than 0.75 mm in thickness) or thick (greater than 0.75 mm). But depth also indicates the seriousness of the melanoma. The deeper and thicker it is, the worse the prognosis.

Many cancer surgeons believe in prophylactic removal of adjacent lymph glands even if none seem to be enlarged upon examination of them. Other surgeons feel that only suspicious lymph glands should be removed. However, despite the use of aggressive surgical, radiological, and chemotherapeutic techniques, malignant melanoma remains a difficult cancer to treat successfully in its advanced stages. Clearly, with a disease like this, early recognition and prompt treatment greatly aid survival rates.

The Sexually Transmitted Diseases

Dermatologists have been involved in the study, diagnosis, and treatment of sexually transmitted diseases (STDs) at least since the nineteenth century. Historically, it was syphilis that really got dermatology into the STD field. This was due in large part to the predominant role the skin symptoms of syphilis played in its early diagnosis. The close connection between dermatology and syphilis is underscored by the fact that beginning in 1914 the main dermatology publication of the American Medical Association was called the *Archives of Dermatology and Syphilology*. Then, in 1950, it was renamed the *Archives of Dermatology*. This reflected a marked decrease in the prevalence of syphilis due to the introduction of penicillin in the 1940s.

The link between dermatology and the diagnosis and treatment of STDs does not, however, just rest on observable skin symptoms. It rests on the fact that the sexual transmission of the STDs are via skin and mucous membrane contact—primarily genital.

And even in those STDs where skin symptoms may not be obvious, the mucous membranes and skin of the genitals are usually affected. However, in this book, I will just discuss the STDs that have the most noticeable skin symptoms. For these are the ones that dermatologists are most likely to diagnose and/or treat.

Different methods are used to diagnose STDs, depending on which particular disease is suspected and what stage the disease is in at the time of diagnosis. Some of these diseases require blood studies to pin down the diagnosis, others depend on laboratory analyses of genital secretions, and some depend on inspection of the skin signs and/or a biopsy of skin tissue.

How do people find out that they have an STD? Sometimes the patient suspects she (or he) has an STD and goes to a doctor to get a diagnosis. Sometimes, however, people come to their doctor with a worrisome sign or symptom but with no suspicion that an STD might be involved. However, with some people and some STDs the symptoms go unnoticed. Especially early symptoms. These are the cases that are either discovered at routine medical checkups by careful and thorough physicians or when the disease has gotten sufficiently advanced that the symptoms become difficult to avoid noticing.

> Knowing the signs and symptoms of the STDs helps you prevent their spread to others and get early treatment for yourself.

The message in all this is to know the signs and symptoms of the STDs and to take great care in their prevention. Although that topic is beyond the scope of this book, you can get helpful information from your local or state public health department. Many run STD hotlines that are listed in your phone book. However, although a number of different methods of protection are available against STDs, abstinence from all sexual contact is the only certain way to avoid contracting these diseases sexually.

Syphilis

Before the introduction of penicillin in the 1940s, syphilis was one of the most ravaging diseases of the twentieth century. Up to fifty percent of most dermatologists' patients had syphilis or one of its complications. However, even with penicillin, syphilis has not been wiped out. There are infected people who are still transmitting it.

The organism that causes the disease is a type of spirochete. Called *Treponema pallidum,* it was first identified in 1905. Shortly thereafter the now famous Wassermann test for syphilis was developed. Since then, a host of blood tests, such as the VDRL, RPR,

STS, and the FTA-ABS, have come onto the scene, each with its own virtues and limitations.

In humans, syphilis goes through three stages—primary, secondary, and tertiary. Each stage is associated with specific skin symptoms.

At the initial, or primary, stage there is the characteristic sore of syphilis—the chancre. It is a .5 to 2 cm sore (about the size of a small blouse button) that appears on the part of the skin that has become infected, usually the genitals. This occurs within a week after exposure. The chancre usually does not hurt or itch or feel tender. Because of anatomical differences in the genitals between women and men, the chancre is easier to see in men. The result of its being so much less observable in women often means that diagnosis takes place at a later stage of the disease than the stage it is caught in men.

> The characteristic skin sign of the primary stage of syphilis—the chancre—fades away after a few weeks even when the disease is still active.

The chancre of the primary stage fades away after a few weeks, even without treatment, as if the problem has resolved. But it has only gone into hiding. In several weeks to months it is followed by the secondary stage. Its symptoms can appear at a number of different places on the body and can assume many different forms, like pustules, bumps, large blotches of redness, or open sores. The skin symptoms of secondary stage syphilis can thus look like any one of a number of different skin conditions. That's why this disease carries the nickname "the great imitator." If left untreated at the secondary stage, progression to tertiary syphilis may occur. The brain, the heart, and the joints are common targets of tertiary syphilis, often with disastrous consequences.

More men than women contract syphilis—it is about six times more common in men as in women. However, this ratio narrows down to two-to-one in late syphilis. The reason for this worsening ratio for women in the later stage of syphilis is as follows. Even though fewer women than men contract it, a greater percentage of men than women get it diagnosed (and thus treated) at the primary stage. This is because the hidden nature of its symptoms in women at the primary stage stands in the way of its early detection. So women go untreated longer and go on to develop more advanced cases. Treatment is the same for both sexes—high doses of penicillin (either intramuscular, at the early stages, or intravenous, in advanced cases).

One thing everyone needs to be aware of is that most people don't think *they* will get syphilis, as if it is a disease that only *other* people get. Once the diagnosis is made, people can be very shocked and their lives can be affected—not just by the disease itself but by the stigma of social attitudes about this illness.

For example, a twenty-year-old woman once walked into my office complaining of hair loss. She was very distraught because she was due to get married in three months. The pattern of hair loss involved patches of baldness mixed together with areas of thinning and areas of fullness. The scalp hair had a moth-eaten appearance.

This patchy hair loss is often a sign of syphilis. Sure enough, the blood test confirmed the diagnosis—it was secondary syphilis.

Humiliated and angered by the diagnosis, the woman requested a repeat test. A more specific test for syphilis gave further confirmation. Fortunately, two shots of penicillin corrected the problem, but the impact of the diagnosis resulted in the marriage being called off despite her full recovery.

Genital Warts (Condyloma Acuminata)

STDs that are caused by viruses are the most difficult to treat, and genital warts is one such disease. (The other prominent viral STD is herpes—discussed below.) Genital warts, known medically as condyloma acuminata, are flesh colored and can be either flat or raised. They do not hurt or itch. Just like regular warts on other parts of the body, genital warts are very contagious.

> STDs, like genital warts and herpes, that are caused by viruses are the most difficult to treat.

Of the fifty different wart viruses that exist, about twelve infect the genital tract. One recent study looked at sexually active adolescent girls aged thirteen to nineteen and found that one out of eight had genital warts.

Many different treatments are available, including topical creams and liquids, freezing, burning, and laser beams. But it is important to keep in mind that warts can be very resistant to treatment. Multiple attempts with different kinds of treatment may be needed. In fact, many physicians feel that genital warts are never 100 percent eradicated and that a small remnant of the virus always lives on microscopically. That is not to say that these warts are incurable, but rather that some people who appear to have been cured may not actually be.

Special attention must be paid to women over the age of forty who have resistant genital warts. It has been found that recurrent condyloma acuminata in this age group may reflect a serious underlying disorder. A report showed that an incredible 38 percent of these women had some kind of an internal cancer. Apparently the body's inability to fight off cancer rendered it more susceptible to the warts as well.

Genital Herpes

Herpes simplex virus type 2 causes another viral STD. It occurs in the genital area. On occasion, albeit with far less frequency, genital herpes can be caused by the herpes simplex virus type 1, the one that causes cold sores, or fever blisters, on the face (see below). Sometimes, genital herpes is also referred to as the "below the belt" type, and the cold sores on the lips, as the "above the belt" type.

Although genital herpes is contagious, regardless of which of the two types of herpes simplex viruses causes it, it is still not as common as genital warts.

Herpes simplex blisters are often preceded by a tingling or burning sensations at the site where they are about to break out.

> **Herpes simplex blisters are often preceded by a tingling or burning sensation.**

There can even be a reddening. Then, sometimes in as little as a few minutes or up to a few days, the blisters appear. The skin at the base of the blisters is red. The fluid in the blisters is quite contagious, meaning that the virus can be transferred by the hands to other parts of the body or to someone else. (Therefore, washing your hands is important after touching an infected area.) Over the next week to ten days, the blisters dry up and disappear, but recurrences in the same area are common.

As with other STDs, women, and men also, may carry the virus and not know they are infected. One study showed that, out of 905 women whose cultures of the genital area tested positive for herpes, only 116 reported having been aware that they had an active genital herpes infection. And when you have one, it is usually hard to miss! They are

> **Though genital herpes is painful, not everyone attributes the pain to herpes—you can have herpes but not know it.**

painful. Apparently, although these women were aware of the pain, they did not attribute it to herpes. But as long as they tested positive for herpes, they could transmit it sexually. So not everyone who is infectious knows they are, and this poses a problem for preventing its spread.

The current treatment for herpes is Zovirax (acyclovir). It comes both as an ointment for topical use and in capsule form to be taken orally. This is the only major drug approved for herpes (although others are being developed). In some people, daily use of this medication may prevent recurrences or dramatically cut down on their frequency, but it is not a cure.

One of the troublesome findings to emerge from data of studies on women with either genital herpes *or* warts is that they have a real danger of developing cervical cancer. Many examples exist in the scientific literature of viruses provoking the growth of cancer. Warts and herpes, through unknown mechanisms, seem to induce changes in the cervix. This change, known as *cervical dysplasia,* can progress into cancer over a number of years. In view of the very high number of women who have asymptomatic infections with either warts or herpes, you can understand the importance of regular gynecologic examinations and Pap smears to detect cancer of the cervix at the earliest possible stage.

Scabies and Lice

Two less common STDs are scabies and lice. Scabies are small mites that pass from person to person on contact. They can be spread sexually and through nonsexual contact (notably among young school children and in the elderly living in nursing homes). The symptoms—small, itchy bumps—may not be apparent until one month after infection. When transmitted sexually, those bumps appear in the genital area initially. Clothing and bedding will often harbor the mite for several days, so that reinfection from contact with fabric in which the mites live is possible even after you and your partner have received the proper treatment.

Lice have a period of incubation similar to scabies, of almost one month. Infected individuals may develop bumps, blisters, and/ or blue spots on the areas where the lice bite. As with scabies, lice can live away from the human body, for example, on bed sheets, for several days. That is why even people who keep clean and who are not sexually active can get lice, and it is also why when treating these conditions, which involves killing the critters and their eggs, such things as

Scabies and lice can live away from the human body—on bed sheets and clothing—for several days.

underwear, bedclothes, hair combs and brushes must be treated. Head lice are generally not transmitted sexually. Pubic lice (often called "crabs") usually, but not always, are.

AIDS (Acquired Immune Deficiency Syndrome)

AIDS is both a sexually and a nonsexually transmitted disease. It has been shown to be caused by the human immunodeficiency virus (HIV, formerly known as HTLV-III). Perfectly healthy, robust people are easily felled by it.

Even as this is written, new information continues to emerge as to when, why, and how the HIV spreads through the body, wreaking havoc with the immune system and causing the person to succumb to many infections. Although the statistics and forecasts regarding AIDS are constantly changing, a number that no one seems to dispute is that the incidence among women is rising rapidly.

Basically the spread of HIV conforms to the following pattern: the bodily fluid of someone infected by the virus—most commonly blood or semen, less often vaginal fluids, and only rarely (if ever) breast milk or saliva—is absorbed into the bloodstream of the previously uninfected person through a break in their outer skin or through a break in the mucous membranes of the vagina, the anus, the mouth, or the conjunctiva of the eyes. The behavior that is most commonly associated with HIV transmission is (1) the sharing of hypodermic needles, often engaged in by users of illicit drugs, where the needles are contaminated with infected blood and (2) unprotected sexual intercourse. Not everyone who is exposed to the virus (either via the sexual route or by nonsexual means) goes on to develop AIDS, but the percentage is quite high.

Dermatologists are often the first to suspect that someone has been infected by HIV. This is because so many of the signs and symptoms of illness associated with HIV—even before it goes on to become AIDS—show up on the skin. The purplish patches of a skin cancer called *Kaposi's sarcoma* (once a rare disease found mostly in elderly men of Mediterranean or Jewish ancestry) were, in fact, one of the first indications that this new disease, AIDS, had come onto the scene: doctors were puzzled when otherwise healthy young men of all ethnic backgrounds started to come in with this unusual skin condition.

Many of the signs and symptoms associated with HIV infection—even before it goes on to become AIDS—show up on the skin.

The link between Kaposi's sarcoma and HIV infection is still very mysterious. So is the relatively low incidence of Kaposi's sarcoma in women as compared to men with HiV.

Compared to their incidence in the general populace certain skin-related infections affect people with HIV or those who have gone on to develop full-blown AIDS with increased frequency. Among these skin infections are both types of herpes, syphilis, canker sores, and yeast (Candida) infections. In women with HIV, yeast infections in the vagina or mouth (thrush) are a very common early sign that HIV is affecting the immune system. Seborrheic dermatitis, a red scaly rash on the face, has been reported in up to 85 percent of AIDS sufferers.

Cold Sores/Fever Blisters

The herpes simplex type 1 virus causes an infection on and around the lips. It is acquired through direct contact with the virus—most usually from someone who has an active herpes type 1 infection, although on rare occasions it can be contracted from contaminated instruments. The blisters are popularly referred to as "fever blisters" or "cold sores." As these terms suggest, the blisters are sometimes associated with fevers and colds, although sun exposure, menstruation, and stress are some of the other factors that precipitate an outbreak.

> The blisters of active herpes type 1 infection are popularly referred to as "fever blisters" or "cold sores."

The virus itself lives within a nerve in the infected area. When you become infected with the herpes simplex type 1 virus, it often doesn't immediately take the active form, but will remain latent until it is triggered. At that point the blisters appear.

The course of the outbreaks is usually three to seven days. Just as with genital herpes simplex infections, cold sores of the lips often start with a tingling sensation and a reddening, followed almost immediately by the characteristic blister.

Recent advances in antiviral therapy have led to the development of acyclovir (Zovirax), a drug that fights the herpes virus. As was discussed in conjunction with the treatment of genital herpes, acyclovir is available as both an oral and topical medication. The oral form can be used for acute attacks or as maintenance (daily) therapy for the prevention of new outbreaks, although it is generally prescribed just for herpes simplex type 2. The topical form of acyclovir is most effective for herpes simplex type 1.

There are currently no drugs that *kill* the herpes simplex virus—acyclovir only suppresses it. That is why it remains latent in the system, emerging periodically as outbreaks of the blisters. In its latent form, skin contact with others cannot transmit the infection.

P*soriasis*

Psoriasis is a common skin disorder that affects approximately 3 percent of the general population. It is characterized by thick white scales that most commonly appear on the elbows, knees, and scalp. It is usually not itchy or painful. Any part of the skin can be affected although the face is usually spared. When the nails are affected they thicken and take on a yellowish color.

Psoriasis is inherited, not contagious, although the exact pattern of inheritance is not well understood. A rare form of psoriasis is called *pustular psoriasis* in which multiple pustules, instead of scales, form. There is also a condition known as *psoriatic arthritis,* which can be very debilitating by deforming the joints.

> **Psoriasis is inherited, not contagious.**

A multitude of therapies exist for psoriasis. Topical steroids, tars, emollients, and ultraviolet treatments are helpful. Powerful drugs, such as methotrexate and etretinate, can also cause psoriasis to go into remission.

S*arcoidosis*

Sarcoidosis, or sarcoid, is a disorder that can affect many systems in the body. It usually occurs in the twenty- to forty-year-old age bracket. Females are affected more than males, and Blacks at a higher frequency than Whites. Skin problems make up a major component of this disease.

Many people get tender red nodules, called erythema nodosum, on the shins. These can actually be the first discernible signs of the disease. Another sign of this condition is lupus pernio—a chronic, purplish bump on the nose, which can progress to ulcerations. (Lupus pernio should not be confused with the collagen vascular disease, lupus, discussed earlier.) Purple patches can appear on the limbs and buttocks. Transient rashes, which can last up to a month, sometimes occur on other parts of the body. Also, scars that were present prior to the onset of sarcoid may become purple and inflamed.

In addition to the skin problems, sarcoidosis frequently involves the lungs. This can be easily determined by a simple chest x-ray. Lymph glands are also affected and may display noticeable swelling. The basic metabolic defect in this illness is a depression in the immune function of the T-cells, whose function is essential to the health of the immune system. Sarcoid responds to immunosuppressive drugs such as high dose steroids and azathioprine.

Anorexia Nervosa and Bulimia

Anorexia nervosa and bulimia are psychiatric and metabolic disorders with well-documented effects on the skin. Anorectics are calorie deprived, with diets that allow them just enough protein to get by. Bulimics ingest all kinds of food, only to self-induce vomiting. Anorectics don't ingest enough calories; bulimics do but vomit them out before they "register" as calories. Anorexia nervosa has been shown to be associated with a decrease in skin thickness as well as in the thickness of subcutaneous fats. This decrease in skin thickness also occurs in other conditions in which there is a prolonged fasting state. And although subsequent weight gain increases subcutaneous fat, it does not increase the skin thickness.

The skin and subcutaneous fat layer become thinner in anorexia nervosa.

Anorectics have been tested to see if their skin has the ability to mount an immune response. A University of Pennsylvania study showed that, like alcoholics, anorectics had a decreased skin immune reaction to Candida (yeast), mumps, and strep. The researchers found that there was a correlation between the degree of malnutrition and the degree of immune loss as indicated by these tests. This is not to say that women with anorexia nervosa are as immune-deficient as persons with AIDS. Unlike in AIDS, where the immune deficiency is the result of the HIV destroying a central part of the immune system, the status of immune deficiency in anorectics is related to their diet.

According to a study in the *Archives of Internal Medicine* most anorectics have surprisingly few infections. Apparently whatever impact their eating deprivations have on their immune system, it does not affect their ability to mount a fight to most infections. This is in striking contrast to AIDS patients.

There are differences between the dietary deficiencies of famine victims and those of anorectics. Famine victims are typically deprived of both protein and calories while anorectics commonly restrict calories in the form of fat and carbohydrates but allow themselves some proteins from vegetables and low-fat cheeses. Thanks to the vegetables in their diet, anorectics are not likely to suffer the severe vitamin deficiencies (and the skin problems that go along with them) common among famine victims. Dry skin with fine scales has been reported in roughly 24 percent of women with anorexia nervosa. This is in keeping with other states of malnutrition. It will probably come as no surprise that vitamin deficiencies can be found in anorectics even though they eat vegetables. And vitamin deficiencies can lead to skin rashes.

There are other skin signs of anorexia nervosa. Cold hands and cold feet are common, and fingers and toes might even be persistently blue. Seventy-two percent of anorectics developed carotenemia—an orange hue to the skin. The reason for this is not fully understood.

> Seventy-two percent of anorectics developed an orange hue to the skin.

A very ominous story was related in the medical journal *Neurology* of a woman who tried to lose weight by taking syrup of ipecac—a powerful gastrointestinal irritant that induces vomiting. Her prolonged use of the medication led to the development of dermatomyositis, a debilitating skin and muscle disease (discussed earlier in this chapter).

The use of diuretics and laxatives, common to anorexia and bulimia, is associated with other skin problems as well. Diuretic use can cause allergic photosensitivity reactions; laxative overuse can produce rashes.

Sometimes, the slightest clue can tip you off to a severe eating disorder. During a routine skin examination of a thin woman in her twenties, I noticed a thickened callus on the knuckle of her right index finger. Only one callus on one knuckle. I suspected bulimia. Here's why. Bulimics lose weight by self-induced vomiting, most frequently initiated by putting their finger down their throats to trigger the gag reflex. Finger gagging often involves an abrasion of the skin against the upper teeth. That is why a callus or persistent sore over just one knuckle, in conjunction with extreme weight loss or low body weight, is a tell-tale diagnostic skin sign in bulimia.

Lyme Disease

A good deal of attention has been given in recent years to a spirochete infection called Lyme disease. The disease, named for an outbreak in Lyme, Connecticut, is transmitted to humans by the bite of a tick. Usually this occurs in and around grassy and wooded areas where people hike and picnic. But people have been bitten in their own back yards. Cases of Lyme disease have been reported from all parts of North America, but predominantly from the Northeast.

The skin can be the earliest marker of this potentially dangerous disease. Large, expanding red rings, known as erythema chronicum migrans, appear on the skin around the bite. The rash is not painful or itchy. Unfortunately, many people who have Lyme disease never show this distinctive "bull's eye" rash, and, for them, diagnosis of the disease then becomes very difficult. (Occasionally the rash also has little bumps.)

If not treated quickly once the symptoms appear, Lyme disease can go on to involve the heart, nervous system, and the joints. Fortunately, early intervention with antibiotics such as tetracycline can bring about a total cure without any further problems, although there are reports of some cases lingering on even with treatment. This has the physicians and researchers who are working with Lyme disease perplexed and concerned, and it is very troubling to those who are afflicted with this condition.

> Early intervention with antibiotics can bring about a total cure of Lyme disease.

But regardless of this, most cases clear up with early treatment. Early treatment, however, requires early diagnosis. And early diagnosis is facilitated if the tick is discovered or the rash is recognized before it disappears. That is not easy. Bites are often either ignored or, if noticed, treated as insignificant medically. But now that this disease has made its appearance, it is no longer wise to be casual about skin bites. This means regular observation for the tiny ticks (which usually cling to the skin for a day or two). This should become a routine health practice if you have been anywhere near trees and grass. Many states' public health and parks departments have helpful literature to enable you to recognize the ticks, remove them safely (try to save the tick in a plastic bag or pill bottle for identification by an expert), and to spot the disease's associated symptoms. If you know or suspect you've been bitten, consult your doctor. And, to reduce the risk of being bitten, protective clothing and the use of insect repellents with the ingredient DEET is very important for any treks into the woods. But don't be lulled into thinking that you can wear casual attire and not use insect repellent to cut the grass on a warm summer's evening in your own back lawn. Unfortunately, ticks can be present there also. Your state may be able to tell you more about this as well.

Hansen's Disease (Leprosy)

Despite the fact that Hansen's disease (leprosy) is one of the oldest known diseases, its exact nature is still not well understood. The organism that causes it is the *Mycobacterium leprae.* The disease is endemic to Asia, although cases can be found almost anywhere in the world. There is no consensus on the issue of just how contagious Hansen's disease is, but it is felt that frequent skin contact with someone who has this disease is necessary for infection to take place.

There are three types of Hansen's disease: *tuberculoid, lepromatous,* and *intermediate.* The tuberculoid form is characterized by a light-colored patch that has decreased sensation to touch and temperature. Nerve damage, especially around the elbow, is common. The more dramatic type of Hansen's disease is the lepromatous type. It can take many different forms—from localized red patches or bumps to widespread ulcers, pigment changes, and noticeable nodules on the face and trunk. The nerves are usually affected, and patients lose sensation in hands and feet. Mental changes are also seen. The intermediate type may have characteristics of both.

The course of Hansen's disease is quite variable. Some cases resolve spontaneously while others, if left untreated, can cause extensive disfigurement.

The most popular drug in the treatment of Hansen's disease is Dapsone, a sulfur derivative. An antituberculosis medication, Rifampin, has also been shown some effectiveness against this disease. Good results have been reported with thalidomide—a drug that had been used as an antinausea agent, but which was banned in the United States during the 1950s due to its association with severe birth defects when used in pregnancy. Before treatments with these drugs were available, people with Hansen's disease were quarantined Now, that is rarely the case.

Less Well-Known Diseases and Conditions That Affect the Skin

The diseases and conditions that follow tend to affect fewer people, and as a result are less well known. They are hardly unimportant, however, since they affect many women and cause considerable suffering. Some of these diseases are quite complex, but in keeping with the spirit of the book, I've concentrated on the signs and symptoms that affect the skin.

Neurofibromatosis (Von Recklinghausen's Disease)

Neurofibromatosis is also known as von Recklinghausen's disease. It is transmitted genetically, with an incidence rate estimated at one per three thousand births. Many of the body's organs are affected, with the skin being quite prominently involved. Soft subcutaneous nodules—called neurofibromas—form. There may be just a few present, but, in extreme cases, the body will be covered with them. These neurofibromas can be very small or very large. Sometimes they affect the nerves, bones, glands, or brain, and cause pain, weakness, and tissue damage. Multiple, flat, coffee-colored spots, called "cafe-au-lait" spots, are also classic signs of this disease, which can occur anywhere on the body.

> Multiple, flat, coffee-colored spots, called "cafe-au-lait" spots, are classic signs of neurofibromatosis.

About 10 percent of the population at large has at least one cafe-au-lait spot, but if a person has at least six such spots greater than 1.5 centimeters in diameter, that is grounds for making the diagnosis of neurofibromatosis. Another sure sign of neurofibromatosis is multiple freckles in the armpits.

Signs and symptoms may begin to appear in childhood. There is no known treatment except to remove the offending neurofibromas. Most people with this condition lead normal, healthy lives.

Albinism

When the pigment-producing cells, the melanocytes, are inactive, the skin and hair lack pigmentation. This condition is called albinism. The people in whom this occurs are referred to as "albinos." Total body albinism is rare and is often associated with eye abnormalities as well. A much more common condition, vitiligo, is described below.

Vitiligo

Sometimes the melanocytes are absent only in certain areas of the body. This is a condition called vitiligo, which is characterized by snowy white patches on the face, hands, feet, or trunk. These skin symptoms are much more noticeable in dark-skinned people. An occasional association between this condition and thyroid disease has been noted. Treatment consists of topical steroids and/or PUVA. The response to treatment is variable.

> Vitiligo is characterized by snowy white patches on the face, hands, feet, or trunk.

Post-Inflammatory Hyperpigmentation

Post-inflammatory hyperpigmentation is a common problem that occurs in Blacks, Asians, Latinos, and in Whites whose skin is olive colored. This condition is due to an abundance of melanin produced in response to skin inflammation of almost any type, like a pimple, burn, or rash. Just as its name suggests, the inflammation leaves a dark spot (the hyperpigmentation), which can last for months or years. Treatment with bleaching creams can be of some benefit. Most recently, laser therapy has been used, with very encouraging results.

> Laser therapy has been used to treat post-inflammatory hyperpigmentation, with very encouraging results.

Sweat Gland (Eccrine Gland) Abnormalities

Several pathologic conditions are manifestations of eccrine gland abnormalities. Heat stroke and heat intolerance occur when the sweat glands cannot keep up with the demands that are placed on the body by conditions of extreme heat, such as high temperatures in the environment or the increase in body temperature produced by vigorous exercise. Excessive sweating or sometimes tight clothing can plug up sweat glands and lead to the formation of miliaria, tiny white pustules commonly found in infants. Certain drugs, such as atropine, which are used to decrease oral secretions, may cause diminished sweating on the skin surface, although it is generally not of any significant importance.

Keratosis Pilaris

A common skin ailment that has female predominance is keratosis pilaris. Tens to hundreds of little, crusty bumps appear on the upper arms. The thighs and cheeks may be affected as well. These bumps actually represent a plugging of the hair follicles. They tend to appear in childhood and fade out at

> In keratosis pilaris, tens to hundreds of little crusty bumps appear on the upper arms.

about forty. The condition can be helped somewhat by the alpha-hydroxy-acids and Retin-A (see chapter 6).

Unilateral Nevoid Telangiectasia (UNT)

Telangiectasia are dilated blood vessels. The small, superficial varicose veins on the thighs and legs, often called "spider veins," are examples of telangiectasia.

Can you imagine a condition where half of your body is covered with telangiectasia? That is just what unilateral nevoid telangiectasia (UNT) is. Small, dilated blood vessels appear on the arm, leg, and trunk of just one side of the body. They stop right at the midline. UNT is thought to be caused by excessive levels of estrogen in the circulation. It is a rare condition seen in pregnancy or in women who take birth control pills. Fortunately, UNT goes away by itself after several months.

Generalized Essential Telangiectasia (GET)

Another rare malady that affects women is called generalized essential telangiectasia (GET). In GET there are many telangiectasia on the arms and legs. These increase in number. Ultimately, the whites of the eyes become involved. As in the case of UNT, GET usually resolves spontaneously with time. The cause is unknown.

Lichen Sclerosus Et Atrophicus (LS&A)

A unique condition that affects the vulva is lichen sclerosus et atrophicus, most often referred to by its initials, "LS&A." This is a chronic disease in which the vulva becomes whitish in color. The mucosa also becomes thinner. Intercourse may become difficult or painful. LS&A may be quite resistant to treatment. It appears to be more common in women who have given birth to one or more children as opposed to those who have never had children. The use of vitamin A or beta-carotene seems to have a preventative effect, although how and why these work still remains to be understood.

Incontinentia Pigmenti (IP)

Incontinentia pigmenti (IP) is an uncommon skin disorder that is seen almost exclusively in women. IP has a very unusual pattern of development. It goes through three stages, which evolve over several years. The initial stage, which appears shortly after birth, consists of lines of blisters on the extremities. These blisters fade out after a few weeks but are replaced by lines of wart-like growths. These warty bumps last for several months. When they disappear, they are followed by swirls of pigmented streaks on the trunk or extremities. These discolorations may last for many years. Problems with the nervous system and eyes are often associated with incontinentia pigmenti. There is no known treatment.

K*eloids*

Keloids are overgrown scars. These scars are thickened tracts of skin that are generally not painful but produce a type of tugging sensation or tightness. They result from the collagen in the skin going wild, usually in reaction to an injury of some sort. The injury can be a cut, a sore, an acne pimple, or a surgical scar. Extensive studies have been done on keloids and why they form, but we have no concrete answers as to what triggers the growth of keloids in any particular person or in response to any particular injury. We do know, however, that for some reason they predominantly occur in Blacks.

> Keloids are overgrown scars that usually are the result of an injury of some sort.

Keloids can be quite disfiguring, especially if they are located on the face. Treatment by excision with a knife, called *cold steel surgery*, is associated with a high recurrence rate and may even aggravate the problem. CO_2 laser excision is felt to be the treatment of choice, although it too may be associated with recurrences. Other options include steroid injections and compression with tight bandages and the application of silicone pads. None of these is a panacea, but they can afford considerable improvement.

A*canthosis* N*igricans*

Acanthosis nigricans occurs in both Whites and Blacks. It is a darkening of the skin that can occur in a variety of circumstances. The actual cause of the increased color is a subtle overgrowth of small skin folds. That is what makes the skin look darker. Just why this overgrowth takes place is unknown. The most common areas affected are the neck and the armpits. Sometimes the darkening is quite subtle as if it could be rubbed off, but sometimes it is quite noticeable. When it occurs around the neck, it has a "ring around the collar" appearance. And although it looks as if you could just scrub it off, alas, this is not the case.

Acanthosis nigricans is seen quite commonly in the obese, fueling the suggestion that weight or perhaps skin rubbing against skin are factors in its development. However, there are a number of other conditions in which acanthosis nigricans is seen, including stomach cancer and thyroid disease. The cause of these associations is unknown.

Ehlers-Danlos Syndrome

Ehlers-Danlos syndrome involves an inherited defect in the collagen formation in the skin, bones, and blood vessels. Eleven different types of Ehlers-Danlos syndrome have been distinguished, each slightly different from the other but involving the same basic defect. Although this disease affects more than the skin, it is the skin that is its predominant target.

The classic symptom of this condition is hyperextensibility of the skin: the skin can be pulled high up and away from the underlying muscles. As a result, the skin can become baggy and bruises easily. Wound healing is impaired since the skin holds together poorly. Wrinkles are common. So are firm calcium deposits underneath the skin. The bones of the body are easily dislocated and joints may become loose: some patients can easily bend back their fingers and touch their forearms. The blood vessels can become very fragile and may tear easily, which is a very serious threat in some cases.

Hidradenitis Suppurativa

Hidradenitis suppurativa is a chronic skin disease affecting the apocrine glands of the armpits and groin areas. The glands in these areas become inflamed and drain pus. Because apocrine glands become active only at puberty, that is when hidradenitis suppurativa is likely to first appear. The persistence of painful, deep nodules and draining pus pockets is a frequent source of embarrassment and discomfort. This condition is seen more commonly in the obese and in people with a tendency towards acne.

Although hidradenitis suppurativa is not a contagious disease, long-term treatment with antibiotics is often necessary.

Although hidradenitis is not a contagious disease, long-term treatment with antibiotics is often necessary. Accutane may be helpful as well but cannot be used in women who are trying to become pregnant or already are.

Pemphigus

Pemphigus is an uncommon but potentially fatal skin disease. It most usually occurs in the sixth and seventh decades of life. Large blisters can form anywhere on the skin or on mucous membranes such as the mouth and genitals. Before cortisone treatments were available the disease was universally fatal. Even today, pemphigus carries somewhat of a risk of death.

Acrodermatitis Enteropathica

This uncommon familial disorder is characterized by a severe blistering and pustular rash around the orifices of the body, especially the mouth, anus, and vagina. In addition, there exists an eczematous type of red, scaly rash on the hands and feet. Occasionally, bald patches will appear on the scalp. Aside from its skin symptoms, people with acrodermatitis enteropathica can have marked diarrhea and gastrointestinal malabsorption. The disease usually shows up within the first year of life and can be fatal if left untreated. Curiously, zinc supplements are the treatment of choice in acrodermatitis enteropathica. A metabolic defect may be its underlying cause.

Hermansky-Pudlak Syndrome

Hermansky-Pudlak syndrome is a rare disease in which there is quite a combination of physiological defects. One is called *oculocutaneous albinism*. This is a loss of pigment in the skin and decreased color in the iris of the eye. In addition, the clotting cells of the blood, known as platelets, are defective, and cuts fail to heal.

Pseudoxanthoma Elasticum

Pseudoxanthoma elasticum involves a degeneration of elastic tissue. As a result, all organs of the body that contain elastic tissue can be affected—the skin, retina, blood vessels, gastrointestinal tract, and the heart. The characteristic symptoms are yellowish pebbles that develop on the neck, armpits, elbows, knees, and 'the abdomen. These small bumps do not itch or bleed, but the skin in the affected area can become thickened or sag. The retina exhibits angioid streaks, which are enlarged blood vessels. The affected elastic tissue of the blood vessels can lead to calcifications, decreased blood supply, and easy rupturing. Therefore, gastrointestinal hemorrhage due to weakened blood vessels is common. These symptoms often do not appear until the childbearing years of life.

Henoch-Schonlein Purpura

Henoch-Schonlein purpura is most commonly found in children but can affect adults as well. The cause is unknown, but it is felt to be due to an immunologic dysfunction or possibly a viral infection. The classic presentation of the disease is the sudden onset of purple patches and bumps on the legs, buttocks, and, sometimes, the arms. These bumps are caused by bleeding in the skin. Bleeding in internal organs such as the gastrointestinal tract and the kidneys can occur as well, leading to hemorrhage and, on rare occasions, death.

Histiocytosis X

Histiocytosis X is actually a generic term for three rare diseases: *Hand-Schuller-Christian disease, Letterer-Siwe disease,* and *eosinophilic granuloma.* The defect these diseases have in common is a proliferation of cells called histiocytes. Any organ of the body can be affected—the most common ones being the lungs, lymph glands, bones, hormone-producing glands, and the skin. The skin effects take the several forms—from flesh-colored bumps to large nodules and ulcerations. The most frequent skin sites are the face and trunk. There is no effective treatment for the disease.

Tuberous Sclerosis

Tuberous sclerosis is an uncommon disorder whose incidence is estimated to be one in thirty thousand births. It was originally known as *Bourneville's disease* and later came to be known as *epiloia,* an acronym for the hallmark features of the disease—*epi*lepsy, *lo*w *i*ntelligence, and *a*denoma sebaceum. The last—adenoma sebaceum—is a skin condition that makes up a major part of the disease. Its symptoms are flesh-colored bumps that congregate around the central portion of the face, almost mimicking a severe case of acne. About 85 percent of patients with tuberous sclerosis are born with one or several white patches on the skin. These are known as "ash-leaf spots," due to their leaf-like configuration. Some of the hairs that make up the eyelashes as well as scalp hairs are white. Pea-sized growths located underneath the ends of the fingernails are another of its characteristics. Also, a patch of thickened skin can often be found on the lower back. This is often referred to as a "shagreen patch." Treatment of the skin signs usually involves removing the unsightly bumps from the face, using the one of the following techniques: excision, lasers, or dermabrasion (discussed in chapter 6).

> The skin symptoms of tuberous sclerosis are flesh-colored bumps that congregate around the central portion of the face.

Glossary ◄

If any terms used in these definitions are unfamiliar, check for them elsewhere in the glossary. If you don't find them, check the index, since many terms are defined within the book.

ablation ▶ The surgical destruction of tissue, as in the removal of a wart or other skin growth.

abrade ▶ To wear down or rub away by friction, as in cosmetic and surgical techniques like dermabrasion and salabrasion.

allergic reaction ▶ A local or general hypersensitivity reaction that involves histamine release from mast cells and can cause inflammation, tissue damage, hives, redness, sneezing, and a variety of other symptoms. *See also* **hypersensitivity**

antibody ▶ A protein produced in the blood or body tissues by the immune system in response to a specific antigen. Antibodies destroy or weaken the antigens.

antigen ▶ A substance, like a bacteria or toxin, that can stimulate the immune system to produce antibodies to fight it.

apocrine glands ▶ Scent glands which, in humans, are found mostly in the underarm and pubic areas. They do not become active until puberty.

areola ▶ The small ring of color around the nipple of the breast.

basal cell layer ▶ The lowest layer of the epidermis. Produces the squamous cells (*see* **squamous cell layer**) and houses the melanocytes.

blanch ▶ To white out, to bleach, to remove color or make pale.

collagen ▶ A fibrous protein found in bone, cartilage, tendons, and connective tissue. It is the backbone of the dermis (the second layer of the skin).

comedogenic ▶ A substance that produces or aggravates acne.

comedone ▶ A plug of keratin and sebum within a hair follicle that is blackened at the surface. It is often referred to as a blackhead.

congenital ▶ Existing at birth, either inherited or due to influences on the fetus while in the womb or at the moment of birth.

cradle cap ▶ A scalp condition that occurs in infants and is characterized by heavy, yellow, crusted lesions.

cross-reaction ▶ The reaction between an antigen and an antibody, but where the antibody developed in reaction to a different although very similar antigen.

curettage ▶ A scraping of the insides of a cavity or of an area of the skin in order to remove growths or other abnormal tissue.

cystic acne ▶ A type of acne where the predominant lesions are cysts and deep-seated scars. (Cysts are membranous sacs containing a semisolid substance.)

dermatitis ▶ Inflammation of the skin.

dermis ▶ The second layer of the skin (right beneath the epidermis). It varies in thickness from one to four millimeters and is thickest on the back of the body and thinnest on the palm of the hand.

desiccate ▶ To dry or burn out.

detergents ▶ A cleaning substance that acts similarly to soap but is made from chemical compounds rather than fats and lye. Detergents are used in shampoos, soaps for the skin, and also in household cleaning products.

eccrine glands ▶ True sweat glands that regulate the body's temperature by delivering water to the skin surface so that heat can be lost by evaporation.

embryo ▶ The prefetal product of conception from the time of implantation of the fertilized egg in the uterus through the eighth week of its development. *See also* **fetus**

emollient ▶ A substance that is softening and soothing to the skin.

endemic ▶ Prevalent or peculiar to a specific locality or people, as in *endemic to the tropics*.

epidermis ▶ Although frequently used as a synonym for *skin*, it is actually the name for its outermost layer only. It is composed of the stratum corneum, the stratum granulosum, the squamous cell layer, and the basal cell layer.

excise ▶ To remove by cutting off or by some other surgical technique, like lasering.

fetus ▶ The unborn young, or product of conception, from the eighth week of development to the moment of birth. *See also* **embryo**

granulomatous ▶ A descriptive term referring to inflamed skin tissue, generally made up of fleshy, beadlike protuberances that often occur in conjunction with healing and infection.

hair follicle ▶ A small cavity or sac on the skin out of which a body hair can grow.

humectant ▶ A substance used to obtain a moistening effect or that promotes the retention of water.

hypersensitivity ▶ A condition of abnormal sensitivity in which there is an exaggerated response by the body to the stimulus of a foreign substance. An allergy is one type of hypersensitivity reaction, but not all hypersensitive reactions are allergic. See *also* **allergic reaction**

inactive ▶ Used to describe chemicals in drug preparations that have no therapeutic effect, although, on occasion, they may have some bodily effect and, on rare occasions, will cause a hypersensitivity reaction.

inert ▶ A substance that doesn't easily (or at all) react with other substances. An inert substance will have no pharmacological (chemical) effect on the body.

inflammation ▶ A localized reaction by body tissue to irritation, and characterized by pain, redness, and/or swelling.

interstitial ▶ The small narrow spaces between tissues or parts of an organ.

keloid ▶ A raised formation of scar tissue caused by excessive tissue repair in response to injury or surgery.

keratin ▶ A tough protein that is a component of skin, hair, and nails.

lentigo ▶ (*pl.* **lentigines**) A small, flat, pigmented spot on the skin.

lesion ▶ Refers (in popular usage and in medicine) to an infected, damaged, or diseased patch of skin. However, in medicine it is also used to refer to any diseased change in a bodily tissue or organ, so that pathology of an internal organ can also be called a lesion.

mast cells ▶ A connective tissue cell that contains histamine, which is released by these cells in allergic reactions. *See* **allergic reaction**

melanocytes ▶ These are cells that make melanin, the skin pigment.

metabolism ▶ The physical and chemical processes that occur in a living cell or organism that are necessary for maintaining life. Also refers to how a specific substance functions. The metabolism of a substance (a drug or a natural biochemical) refers to the changes it goes through as the body's physiological processes affect it.

mole ▶ *See* **nevus**

mucous membrane ▶ A thin layer of pliable tissue that lines a body cavity, like the mouth or vagina, and is covered by a clear, thick, sticky secretion.

nevus ▶ (*pl.* **nevi**) A benign localized growth of cells of the skin, commonly known as a mole. May be flat or raised, and usually is dark in color.

palmar warts ▶ Warts on the palm of the hand.

pathology ▶ The anatomical, physiological, or functional manifestation of disease.

placebo ▶ A substance with no known beneficial effect that is presented as if it is a medication that has potentially beneficial effects. Generally given to a control group in scientific experiments to compare the outcomes of the control group with the test group (the group that is given the medicine) in order to determine if any results are due to the *belief* that the substance given might be an effective drug or due to the actual physiologic effects of the drug being tested. *See also* **placebo effect**

placebo effect ▶ Refers to a beneficial effect derived from getting a substance that has no known medicinal effect but is believed to be potentially therapeutic. The mind-body mechanism of how this works is not well understood.

pruritus ▶ Severe itching of the skin.

pustule ▶ A small elevation on the skin that contains pus.

receptor ▶ A specialized cell or group of nerve endings that responds to sensory stimuli or binds (unites or coheres) with substances like hormones, drugs, and other biochemicals.

scar ▶ A mark left on the skin after an injury to skin tissue has healed.

sebaceous glands ▶ Oil glands attached to hair follicles. These glands are found everywhere on the skin except the palms of the hands and the soles and tops of the feet.

sebum ▶ A semifluid secretion of the sebaceous glands, made up chiefly of fat, keratin, and cellular material.

sclerosis ▶ A thickening or hardening of part of the body, like an artery, especially from fibrous interstitial tissue.

sign ▶ An abnormality that indicates disease (pathology) that is discoverable by examination. An example of a sign is a bump on the skin. Another is an enlarged spleen. *See also* **symptom**

slough ▶ To shed or to separate away from surrounding living tissue.

SPF ▶ *See* **sun protection factor**

squamous cell layer ▶ The third layer of the epidermis, which lies between the stratum granulosum and the basal cell layer (the lowest layer of the epidermis). The cells that make up the squamous cell layer are the most abundant cells of the skin and function as a transport medium for water.

stratum corneum ▶ The outer coating of the epidermis. It consists of compacted dead cells called keratin, which is a dried-out protein. Also called the **horny layer.**

stratum granulosum ▶ The layer of the epidermis that lies beneath the stratum corneum. Also called the **granular layer.**

subcutaneous layer ▶ The innermost layer of the skin (right beneath the dermis). It is composed of fat, and in most areas of the skin, it is thicker than the dermis. It serves as an insulator in order to conserve body heat and functions as a shock absorber to protect the internal organs against trauma.

sun protection factor ▶ The numerical value assigned to a sunscreen based on its ability to protect against sunburn. *Also known as* **SPF.**

symptom ▶ An experience of an irregular or painful sensation or change in the structure and function in some aspect of the body. *See also* **sign**

toxic ▶ A chemical substance that is poisonous (destructive) and can cause injury to bodily tissue and, in some cases, death.

vulva ▶ The external part of a woman's genitals, including the labia, clitoris, and the outer part of the vagina.

Organizations ◄

▶ American Academy of Family Physicians
8880 Ward Parkway, Kansas City, MO 64114
(816) 333-9700

▶ American Academy of Pediatrics
141 Northwest Point Blvd., P.O. Box 927,
Elk Grove Village, IL 60009-0927
(708) 228-5005

▶ American Anorexia/Bulimia Association
418 E. 76th St., New York, NY 10021
(212) 734-1114

▶ American Cancer Society
1599 Clifton Rd. N.E., Atlanta, GA 30329
(404) 320-3333

▶ American College of Obstetricians and Gynecologists
409 12th St. S.W., Washington, DC 20024-2188
(202) 638-5577

▶ American Dietetic Association
216 W. Jackson Blvd., Suite 800, Chicago, IL 60606-6995
(312) 899-0040

▶ American Foundation for the Prevention of Venereal Disease
799 Broadway, Suite 638, New York, NY 10003
(212) 759-2069

▶ American Geriatrics Society
770 Lexington Ave., Suite 300, New York, NY 10021
(212) 308-1414

▶ American Medical Association
515 N. State St., Chicago, IL 60610
(312) 464-5000

▶ American Medical Women's Association
801 N. Fairfax St., Suite 400, Alexandria, VA 22314
(703) 838-0500

▶ American Osteopathic Association
142 E. Ontario St., Chicago, IL 60611
(312) 280-5800

▶ American Psychological Association
750 1st St. N.E., Washington, DC 20002
(202) 336-5500

▶ American Nurses Association
2420 Pershing Rd., Kansas City, MO 64108
(816) 474-5720

▶ American Social Health Association
P.O. Box 13827, Research Triangle Park, NC 27709
(919) 361-8400

▶ Anorexia Nervosa and Related Eating Disorders
P.O. Box 5102, Eugene, OR 97405
(503) 344-1144

▶ Cosmetic, Toiletry and Fragrance Association
1101 17th St. N.W., Suite 300, Washington, DC 20036
(202) 331-1770

▶ Ehlers Danlos National Foundation
P.O. Box 1212, Southgate, MI 48195
(313) 282-0180

▶ Federation of Feminist Women's Health Centers
633 E. 11th Ave., Eugene, OR 97401
(503) 344-0966

▶ International Association of Trichologists
37320 22nd St., Kalamazoo, MI 49009
(616) 372-3224

▶ Lupus Erythematosus Support Club
8039 Nova Ct., North Charleston, SC 29420
(803) 764-1769

▶ Lupus Foundation of America
4 Research Place, Ste. 180, Rockville, MD 20850
(301) 670-9292 [business line]// (800) 558-0121 [info line]

▶ NAACOG: *The Organization for Obstetric, Gynecologic and Neonatal Nurses*
700 14th St N.W., Washington, DC 20005
(202) 662-1600

▶ *National AIDS Information Clearinghouse*
P.O. Box 6003, Rockville, MD 20849-6003
(301) 217-0023

▶ *National Alopecia Areata Foundation*
710 C St., Suite 11, San Rafael, CA 94901
(415) 456-4644

▶ *National Anorexic Aid Society*
445 E. Granville Rd., Worthington, OH 43085
(614) 436-1112

▶ *National Association of Anorexia Nervosa and Associated Eating Disorders*
Box 7, Highland Park, IL 60035
(708) 831-3438

▶ *National Association of Pediatric Nurse Associates and Practitioners*
1101 Kings Highway N., Ste. 206, Cherry Hill, NJ 08034
(609) 667-1773

▶ *National Association of School Nurses*
P.O. Box 1300, Scarborough, ME 04070-1300
(207) 883-2117

▶ *National Federation of Licensed Practical Nurses*
1418 Aversboro Rd., Garner, NC 27529
(919) 779-0046

▶ *National Neurofibromatosis Foundation*
141 5th Ave., Suite 7S, New York, NY 10010-7105
(212) 460-8980

▶ *National Organization for Rare Disorders*
P.O. Box 8923, New Fairfield, CT 06812
(203) 746-6518

▶ *National Vitiligo Foundation*
P.O. Box 6337, Tyler, TX 75711
(903) 534-2925

▶ *National Women's Health Network*
1325 G St. N.W., Washington, DC 20005
(202) 347-1140

▶ *National Women's Health Resource Center*
2440 M St. N.W., Suite 325, Washington, DC 20037
(202) 293-6045

▶ *Obsessive Compulsive Foundation*
P.O. Box 70, Milford, CT 06460
(203) 878-5669

▶ *Scleroderma Federation*
Peabody Office Bldg., One Newbury St., Peabody, MA 01960
(508) 535-6600

▶ *Scleroderma Federation of the Tri-State Area*
1182 Teaneck Rd., Teaneck, NJ 07666
(201) 837-9826

▶ *Skin Cancer Foundation*
245 5th Ave., Suite 2402, New York, NY 10016
(212) 725-5176

Bibliography ◄

▶ **General**

Boston Women's Health Book Collective. *The New Our Bodies, Ourselves: A Book By and For Women* (New York: Simon & Schuster, Inc., 1992).

Fitzpatrick, T. B. et al. *Dermatology in General Medicine.* New York: McGraw-Hill, 1979.

Parrish, J. A. *Dermatology and Skin Care.* New York: McGraw-Hill, 1975.

▶ **Women's Skin, Men's Skin—What's The Difference?**

Berardesca, E. et al. "Skin Extensibility Time in Women. Changes in Relation to Sex Hormones." *Acta Dermato-Venereologica* 69 (1987): 431–433.

Escoffier, C. et al. "Age-related Mechanical Properties of Human Skin: An *In Vivo* Study." *Journal of Investigative Dermatology* 3 (1989): 353–357.

Graham, T. E. et al. "Thermal and Metabolic Responses to Cold by Men and by Eumenorrheic Women." *Journal of Applied Physiology* 67 (1) (1989): 282–290.

Kolka, M. A., and L. A. Stephenson. "Control of Sweating during the Human Menstrual Cycle." *European Journal of Applied Physiology and Occupational Physiology* 58 (1989): 890–895.

Lammintausta, K. et al. "Irritant Reactivity in Males and Females." *Contact Dermatitis* 17 (1987): 276–280.

Nunneley, S. "Physiological Responses of Women to Thermal Stress: A Review." *Medicine and Science in Sports and Exercise* 10 (4) (1978): 250–255.

Robert C. et al. "Study of Skin Ageing as a Function of Social and Professional Conditions: Modification of the Rheological Parameters Measured with a Noninvasive Method—Identometry." *Gerontology* 34 (1988): 284–290.

▶ **Basics**

Alvarez, L. C. et al. "Changes in the Epidermis during Prolonged Fasting." *American Journal of Clinical Nutrition* 28 (1975): 866–871.

Black, M. M., E. Bottoms, and S. Shuster. "Skin Collagen Thickness in Simple Obesity." *British Medical Journal* 4 (1971): 149–150.

Bourne, S., and A. Jacobs. "Observations on Acne, Seborrhea and Obesity." *British Medical Journal* 34 (1956): 1268.

Davies, C.T.M. et al. "Temperature Regulation in Anorexia Nervosa Patients during Prolonged Exercise." *Acta Medica Scandinavica* 205 (1979): 257–262.

Gupta, M. A. et al. "Dermatologic Signs in Anorexia Nervosa and Bulimia Nervosa." *Archives of Dermatology* 123 (1987): 1386–1390.

Kirby, S. L., and F. L. Iber. "Decreased Hair Pulling Pressure and Impaired Skin Hypersensitivity—Common Abnormal Nutritional Parameters in Alcoholics." *American Journal of Clinical Nutrition* 33 (1980): 937.

Pochi, P. E., D. T. Downing, and J. S. Strauss. "Sebaceous Gland Response in Man to Prolonged Total Caloric Deprivation." *Journal of Investigative Dermatology* 55 (5) (1970): 303–309.

▶ Skin and the Life Cycle

Kligman, A. M. "Postadolescent Acne in Women." *Cutis* 46 (1) (1991): 75–81.

Kligman, A. M. "Postmenopausal Acne." *Cutis* 46 (5) (1991): 425–428.

Schachner, L. A. "Dermatologists Should Be Alert to Cutaneous Signs of Child Abuse." *Dermatology Times* 13 (4) (1992): 1.

▶ The Skin in Pregnancy

Berde, C., D. C. Willis, and E. C. Sandberg. "Pregnancy in Woman with Pseudoxanthoma Elasticum." *Obstetrics and Gynecology* 38 (6) (1983): 339–344.

Burton, J. L. et al. "Effect of Pregnancy on Sebum Secretion." *British Medical Journal* 2 (1970): 769–771.

Hellreich, P. D. "The Skin Changes of Pregnancy." *Cutis* 13 (1974): 82–86.

Hewitt, D. and R. Hillman. "Relation between Rate of Nail Growth in Pregnant Women and Estimated Previous General Growth Rate." *American Journal of Clinical Nutrition* 19 (1966): 436.

Jick, S. et al. "First Trimester Tretinoin and Congenital Disorders." *Lancet* 341 (1993): 1181–1182.

Koren, G. and M. Bologa. "Teratogenic Risk of Hair Care Products." *JAMA* 262 (20) (1989): 2925.

Lynfield, Y. L. "Effect of Pregnancy on the Human Hair Cycle." *Journal of Investigative Dermatology* 35 (1960): 323.

McCoy, M. "Henoch-Schonlein Purpura and Pregnancy." *American Journal Obstetrics and Gynecology* 141 (4) (1981): 469–470.

McKenzie, A. W. "Skin Disorders in Pregnancy." *Practitioner* 206 (1971): 733–780.

Marks, R. "Porphyria Cutanea Tarda." *Archives of Dermatology* 118 (1982): 452.

Mattison, D. R. "Transdermal Drug Absorption during Pregnancy." *Clinical Obstetrics and Gynecology* 33 (4) (1990): 718–727.

Ogburn, P. L. et al. "Histiocytosis X and Pregnancy." *Obstetrics and Gynecology* 58 (4) (1981): 513–515.

Plauche, W. C. "Henoch-Schonlein Neuropathy in Pregnancy." *Obstetrics and Gynecology* 56 (4) (1980): 515–519.

Rattan, P. K. et al. "Tuberous Sclerosis in Pregnancy." *Obstetrics and Gynecology* 62 (1983): 21S–22S.

Reece, E. A. et al. "Tuberous Sclerosis in Pregnancy." *Obstetrics and Gynecology* 57 (1) (1981): 467–468.

Reiss, R. E. et al. "Hermansky-Pudlak Syndrome in Pregnancy: Two Case Studies." *American Journal of Obstetrics and Gynecology* 153 (1985): 564–565.

Riberti, C. et al. "Malignant Melanoma: The Adverse Effect of Pregnancy." *British Journal of Plastic Surgery* 34 (1981): 338–339.

Rothman, K. F., and P. E. Pochi. "Use of Oral and Topical Agents for Acne in Pregnancy." *Journal of the American Academy of Dermatology* 19 (3) (1988): 431–442.

Spiera, H. "The Clinical Picture of Connective Tissue Diseases in Pregnancy." In *Reproductive Immunology*, pp. 303–307. New York: Alan R. Liss, Inc., 1981.

Verburg, D. J. et al. "Acrodermatitis Enteropathica and Pregnancy." *Obstetrics and Gynecology* 44 (2) (1974): 233–237.

Winton, G. B., and C. W. Lewis. "Dermatoses of Pregnancy." *Journal of the American Academy of Dermatology* 6 (1982): 977–998.

Wong, R. E., and C. N. Ellis. Physiologic Skin Changes in Pregnancy." *Journal of the American Academy of Dermatology* 10 (6) (1984): 929–940.

Zilliagus, H. "Porphyria and Pregnancy." *Annales Chirurgiae et Gynaecologiae Fenniae* 56 (1967): 349–353.

▶ Cleanliness, Care, and Cosmetics

Abdelaziz, A. A. et al. "Microbial Contamination of Cosmetics and Personal Care Items in Egypt—Eye Shadows, Mascaras, and Face Creams." *Journal of Clinical Pharmacy and Therapeutics* 14 (1989): 21–28.

Abdelaziz, A. A. et al. "Microbial Contamination of Cosmetics and Personal Care Items in Egypt—Shaving Creams and Shampoos." *Journal of Clinical Pharmacy and Therapeutics* 14 (1989): 29–34.

Caravati, E. M., and T. L. Litovitz. "Pediatric Cyanide Intoxication and Death from an Acetonitrile-containing Cosmetic." *JAMA* 260 (23) (1988): 3470–3473.

Dermatology Times staff. "Blemish Treatments." *Dermatology Times* (Jan. 1992):36.

Dermatology Times staff. "Sunscreen Myths." *Dermatology Times* (Jan. 1992):41.

Fisher, A. A. "Cosmetic Actions and Reactions: Therapeutic, Irritant and Allergic." *Cutis* 26 (1980): 22.

Fisher, A. A. "Cosmetic Warning: This Product May Be Detrimental to Your Purse." *Cutis* 39 (1987): 23–24.

Givens, A. "Home remedies." *Skin and Allergy News* (Feb. 1992):4.

Jackson, E. M. "An In-depth Analysis of Moisturizers." *Cosmetic Dermatology* 12 (1991): 39–42.

Johnson, B. A. "Requirements in Cosmetics for Black Skin." *Dermatologic Clinics* 6 (3) (1988): 489–492.

Lazar, P. "Cosmetics, Barnum, and Science." *Cutis* 39 (1987): 335–336.

Matsuoka, L. Y. et al. "Skin Types and Epidermal Photosynthesis of Vitamin D_3." *Journal of the American Academy of Dermatology* 23 (3) (1990): 525–526.

Mills, O. H. and A. M. Kligman. "Evaluation of Abrasives in Acne Therapy." *Cutis* 23 (1979): 704.

Pacher, F. "Adverse Reactions to Eye Area Cosmetics and Their Management." *Journal of the Society of Cosmetic Chemists* 33 (1982): 249.

Patel, N. P., A. Highton, and R. L. Moy. "Properties of Topical Sunscreen Formulations." *Journal of Dermatologic Surgery and Oncology* 18 (1992): 316–320.

▶ Medical and Surgical Approaches to Cosmetic Problems

Wrinkles and Age Spots

Daniell, H. W. "A Study of the Epidemiology of 'Crow's Feet.'" *Annals Internal Medicine* 75 (1971): 873–880.

Ellis, D. A. and H. Masri. "The Effect of Facial Animation on the Aging Upper Half of the Face." *Archives of Otolaryngology—Head and Neck Surgery* 115 (1989): 710–713.

Pinski, K. S. and H. H. Roenigk. "Autologous Fat Transplantation, Long-Term Follow-up." *Journal of Dermatologic Surgery and Oncology* 18 (1992): 179–184.

Retin-A

Bazzano, G. S. "Topical Tretinoin for Hair Growth Promotion." *Journal of the American Academy of Dermatology* 15 (4) (1986): 880–883.

Burke, K. E., and G. F. Graham. "Tretinoin for Photoaging Skin: North Carolina vs. New York." *JAMA* 260 (21) (1988): 3130–3131.

Chytil, F. "Retinoic Acid: Biochemistry and Metabolism." *Journal of the American Academy of Dermatology* 15 (4) (1986): 741–747.

Goldfarb, M. T. et al. "Topical Tretinoin Therapy: Its Use in Photoaged Skin." *Journal of the American Academy of Dermatology* 21 (3) (1989): 645–650.

Haas, A. A., and K. A. Arndt. "Selected Applications of Topical Tretinoin." *Journal of the American Academy of Dermatology* 15 (4) (1986): 870–877.

Hogan, D. J. "Scarring Following Inappropriate Use of 0.05% Tretinoin Gel." *Journal of the American Academy of Dermatology* 17 (6) (1987): 1056–1057.

Kamm, J. J. "Toxicology, Carcinogenicity, and Teratogenicity of Some Orally Administered Retinoids." *Journal of the American Academy of Dermatology* 6 (4) (1982): 652–659.

Kligman, A. M. "Guidelines for the Use of Topical Tretinoin (Retin-A) for Photoaged Skin." *Journal of the American Academy of Dermatology* 21 (3) (1989): 650–654.

Kligman, A. M. et al. "Topical Tretinoin for Photoaged Skin." *Journal of the American Academy of Dermatology* 15 (4) (1986): 836–858.

Kripke, M. L., and H. N. Glassman. "Retinoic Acid and Photocarcinogenesis Workshop." *Journal of the American Academy of Dermatology* 2 (5) (1980): 439–442.

Lowe, N. et al. "General Discussion of Articles on Tretinoin." *Journal of the American Academy of Dermatology* 15 (4) (1986): 785–788.

Posey, R. A. "Improvement in Old Areas of Radiodermatitis by Using Retin-A Cream." *Schoch Letter* 40 (5) (1990): 18–19.

Shalita, A. "Retin-A for Wrinkles; Daily Use Preferred." *Skin Allergy News* 21 (3) (1990): 1, 14.

Stuttgen, G. "Historical Perspectives of Tretinoin." *Journal of the American Academy of Dermatology* 15 (4) (1986): 735–740.

Weiss, J. S. et al. "Topical Tretinoin Improves Photoaged Skin. *JAMA* 259 (4) (1988): 527–532.

Alpha-Hydroxy-Acids

Dial, W. F. "Use of AHAs Adds New Dimensions to Chemical Peeling." *Cosmetic Dermatology* 5 (1990): 32–34.

Pinnell, S. R. et al. "Induction of Collagen Synthesis by Ascorbic Acid." *Archives of Dermatology* 123 (6) (1987): 1684–1686.

Van Scott, E. J. "Dry Skin et Cetera, Corneocyte Detachment, Desquamation and Neo-strata." *International Journal of Dermatology* 26 (2) (1987): 90.

Van Scott, E. J. and R. J. Yu. "Alpha-Hydroxy-Acids: Procedures for Its Use in Clinical Practice." *Cutis* 43 (1989): 222–228.

Van Scott, E. J. and R. J. Yu. "Control of Keratinization with Alpha-Hydroxy-Acids and Related Compounds." *Archives of Dermatology* 110 (4) (1974): 586–590.

Van Scott, E. J. and R. J. Yu. "Hyperkeratinization, Corneocyte Cohesion, and Alpha-Hydroxy-Acids." *Journal of the American Academy of Dermatology* 11 (5) (1984): 867–879.

Wonder Creams That Never Made It

Brown, G. L. et al. "Enhancement of Wound Healing by Topical Treatment with Epidermal Growth Factor." *New England Journal of Medicine* 321 (2) (1989): 76–79.

Edwards, L., N. Levine, and K. A. Smiles. "The Effect of Topical Interferon Alpha$_{2b}$ on Actinic Keratoses." *Journal of Dermatologic Surgery and Oncology* 16 (1990): 446–449.

Natow, A. J. "Aloe Vera, Fact or Fiction." *Cutis* 37 (1986): 106–108.

Stadler, R. et al. "Interferons in Dermatology." *Journal of the American Academy of Dermatology* 20 (4) (1989): 650–656.

Wehr, R. F., and L. Krochmal. "Considerations in Selecting a Moisturizer." *Cutis* 39 (1987): 512–515.

▶ The Hair and Nails

Barth, J. H. et al. "Spironolactone in an Effective and Well-tolerated Systemic Antiandrogen Therapy for Hirsute Women." *Journal of Clinical Endocrinology and Metabolism* 68 (4) (1989): 966–969.

Brauer, E. W. "Selected Prostheses Primarily of Cosmetic Interest." *Cutis* 6 (1970): 521.

Guttman, C. "Many Nail Disorders Occupation-related." *Dermatology Times* 13 (2) (1992): 52.

Hochman, L. G. et al. "Brittle Nails: Response to Daily Biotin." *Cutis* 1 (1993): 303–305.

March, C. H. "Allergic Contact Dermatitis to a New Formula to Strengthen Nails." *Archives of Dermatology* 93 (1966): 270.

Marks, J. F., M. E. Bishop, and W. P. Willis. "Allergic Contact Dermatitis to Sculptured Nails." *Archives of Dermatology* 115 (1979): 100.

Martikainen, H. et al. "Hormonal and Clinical Effects of Ketoconazole in Hirsute Women." *Journal of Clinical Endocrinology and Metabolism* 66 (5) (1988): 987–999.

Morrison, L. H., and F. J. Storrs. "Persistence of an Allergen in Hair after Glyceryl Monothioglycolate-containing Permanent Wave Solutions." *Journal of the American Academy of Dermatology* 19 (1988): 52.

Venning, V. A., and R.P.R. Dawber. "Patterned Androgenic Alopecia in Women." *Journal of the American Academy of Dermatology* 18 (5) (1988): 1073–1077.

Wilborn, W. S. "Black Women Risk Injury from Hair Restructuring Products." *Dermatology Times* (Sept. 1991):6.

▶ Other Skin Conditions, Diseases, and Reactions

Carmichael, J. A., and P. D. Maskens. "Cervical Dysplasia and Human Papillomavirus." *American Journal of Obstetrics and Gynecology* 160 (1989): 916–918.

Kjaer, S. K. et al. "Human Papillomavirus, Herpes Simplex Virus, and Cervical Cancer Incidence in Greenland and Denmark. A Population-based Cross-sectional Study." *International Journal of Cancer* 41 (1988): 518–524.

Koening, K. L. "Hair Dye Use and Breast Cancer." *American Journal of Epidemiology* (133 (10) (1991): 985–995.

Marshburn, P. B., and K. F. Trofatter. "Recurrent Condyloma Acuminatum in Women over Age 40: Association with Immunosuppression and Malignant Disease." *American Journal of Obstetrics and Gynecology* 159 (1988): 429–433.

Martin, K. L. "Genital Herpes Virus May Be Asymptomatic." *Modern Medicine* 57 (1989): 11.

Martinez, J. et al. "High Prevalence of Genital Tract Papillomavirus Infection in Female Adolescents." *Pediatrics* 82 (4) (1988): 604–608.

eccrine glands, 12–13, 14, 36, 50, 62–63, 236; abnormalities of, 227
eczema, 34–35, 121; dyshidrotic, 63; xerotic, 47
edema, 47
Ehlers-Danlos syndrome, 80–81, 230
elastic fibers, 12, 135; degeneration of, 231
elasticity of skin, 2–3, 15, 49, 63–64
electrodesiccation. See desiccation
electrolysis, 196
embryo, 236
embryocidal substances, 56
emollient, 236
emphysema, symptoms of, in nails, 201
endemic, defined, 236
enzymes, 12
eosinophilic granuloma, 232
epidermis, 10–11, 236; in fasting, 21; Retin-A's effect on, 114, 128; thinned by AHAs, 134
epidermolysis, 134
epidermolytic hyperkeratosis, 122
epilation, electrical. See electrolysis
epilepsy, 232
epiloia, 232
Epsilon-aminocaproic acid, 149
Epstein, Dr. John, 128–129
erythema, palmar, 66
erythema chronicum migrans, 224
erythromycins, 58, 73
estradiol, 49
estrogen, 4, 5, 10, 63, 169; and acne, 72; in birth control pills, 42, 83; contraindicated during pregnancy and breastfeeding, 58, 60; and gums, 67; and hirsutism, 195; moles affected by, 74; stimulates melanocytes and melanomas, 61, 77
estrogen therapy, 49; and hair loss, 193, 194
etretinate, 73, 221
excision, 67, 78, 151, 163, 211, 229, 233, 236
exercise, and heat tolerance, 4
extensibility of skin, 6, 15
eyelashes, artificial, 107
eyelids, sagging, 171–173
eyeliner, 107

eye makeup, 106–107
eye shadow, 104

face lifts, 8, 110, 149, 154, 157–158, 162, 178; side effects of, 158–159
face peels. See peels
facial cosmetics, 105–107
facial treatments, 178
facial veins, removal of, 169–171
fade creams, 108
famine victims, 222–223
fashion, gendered skin differences and, 6–8
fasting, 21
fat, 3, 12; consumption of, 21. See also liposuction; lipoinjection
FDA risk categories, for drug use in pregnancy, 55–57
feet, occupational problems of, 207–208
fetus, 5, 13, 53, 54, 57, 236; abnormalities in, 38 (see also birth defects); and Accutane, 73; and dermatomyositis, 79; and impetigo herpetiformis, 86; and lupus, 78; and mother's immune system, 71; and Spangler's dermatitis, 86, 87; STDs as risk to, 75–76; tetracycline's effect on, 58
fever blisters, 34, 75–76, 153, 217, 220–221
Fibrel, 149–150
Fields, W. C., 156
fifties, skin conditions of persons in their, 46–49
filler substances, injectible, 147–150
fingernails, 17–18
finger warts, 30
5-fluoro-uracil (5-FU), 51, 145–146
flushing, during menopause, 49
follicles, hair, 13, 16–17, 151, 193, 227, 236
Food and Drug Administration. See FDA risk categories
formaldehyde, 189
forties, skin conditions of persons in their, 44–46
foundations, cosmetic, 105, 106, 185
Fox-Fordyce disease, 14
fragrance, 104
freckles, 74, 108, 121

130; use of, 121–124; Voorhees's study of, 112–114, 116, 125
retinol, 117. *See also* vitamin A
rhinophyma, 156
riboflavin, 18
rifampin, 79–80, 225
ringworm, 33, 192
risk categories, FDA, for drug use in pregnancy, 55–57
Roberts, Julia, 162
Rogaine, 69, 193–194
rosacea, 44–45, 156, 169
Rothman, Dr. Karen, 127
rouge, facial, 105, 185
rubber. *See* latex
rubella (German measles), 33, 89
ruby laser, 164–165

sagging eyelids, 171–173
salabrasion, 164
salicylic acid, 94; soaps, 91
salt, table. *See* sodium chloride
sarcoidosis, 80, 221–222
sarcosines, 182
scabies, 218
scalp, 16, 33, 68, 182, 183, 193
scarring, 237; from acne, 148, 151, 154–155, 162, 175, 178–179; from electrolysis, 196; from excessive use of Retin-A, 126; hypertrophic, 156–157; from tattoo removal, 164; traumatic, 155;. *See also* keloids
Schachner, Dr. Lawrence, 28
science, normal, procedures and methodology of, 2, 55, 112–114, 116
scleroderma, 79, 180, 210
sclerosis, 237
sclerotherapy, 65, 166–167; side effects from, 167–169
scopolamine, 10
sculptured nails, 190–191
scurvy, 18, 68
sebaceous glands, 12, 13, 49, 151, 237
sebaceous hyperplasia, 45–46
seborrheic dermatitis, 220
seborrheic keratosis, 43–44, 50, 136, 212
sebum, 237. *See also* oil, skin
serum lipids, 38
sex differences in skin, 1–8

sexual abuse, child, 29
sexually transmitted diseases (STDs), 4, 213–220; and pregnancy, 75–77
Shalita, Dr. Alan, 125
shampoos, 181–183; antifungal, 39–40; side effects of, 183–184
shaving, 6, 195
"shiners": allergic, 35; from blepharoplasty, 172
shingles, 34
shivering, 10
shoes, allergic reactions to dyes in, 205
sign, of malady, defined, 238. *See also* symptom
silicone injections, 180
sixties and up, skin conditions of persons in their, 49–52
skin: allergic reactions of, 204–205; "alligator" (*see* ichthyosis); basal cell layer, 11, 235; blood circulation and, 47; cancers of, 25, 40, 43, 44, 50, 98, 140–141, 210–213 (*see also* basal cell carcinoma; Kaposi's sarcoma; malignant melanoma; squamous cell carcinoma); characteristics of, 14–15; cleanliness of, 90–94; color, natural, 11 (*see also* pigmentation); dermis (*see* dermis); dry, 133, 136, 197; elasticity of, 2–3, 49, 63–64; epidermis (*see* epidermis); external temperature and, 3–4; function of, 9–10; gender differences in, 1–8; grafting, 163, 178; granular layer, 10, 238 (*see also* skin: stratum corneum); and human life cycle, 24–26; hyperextensibility of, 80–81; layers of, 10–12; mucous membrane, 4, 213–214, 219, 237; nutrition and, 18–23 (*see also* anorexia nervosa); occupational disorders of, 205, 206, 207–208; over-the-counter preparations and personal care products, 94–98, 101–103; precancerous conditions of, 25, 40, 43, 44, 50, 98, 140–141, 165 (*see also* actinic keratoses; moles); pre-existing conditions, and pregnancy, 71–84; pregnancy's effects on,

David M. Stoll, M.D., is a board-certified dermatologist in private practice in Beverly Hills, California. He went to medical school and did his dermatology residency at Vanderbilt University Medical Center. Dr. Stoll is a Fellow of the American Academy of Dermatology. He has a special interest in laser and cosmetic surgery.